The Healer Within

Achieving Optimum Health With
Empowering Habits, Emotional
Freedom, and the Miracle of CBD Oil

By William Pieper

Literary Contributor, Stella Gimenez

Editor, Brian M. F. Burch

i

DISCLAIMER

The contents of this book, all text, graphics, images, studies and information are for informational purposes only. This book does not intend as a substitute for the medical advice of physicians. Neither to prevent, alleviate, or cure any disease or disorder. For diagnosis or treatment of any medical problem, consult your physician. The publisher and author are not responsible for any specific health or allergy needs that may require medical supervision. They are not liable for any damages or negative consequences from any treatment, action, application or preparation, to any person reading or following the information in this book. References we provide here are for informational purposes only and do not constitute an endorsement of any websites or other sources. Readers should be aware that the websites listed in this book may change. The reader should regularly consult a physician in matters relating to his/her health, and particularly with respect to any symptoms that may require diagnosis or medical attention.

Always check with your physician before starting a new dietary supplement program. The Food and Drug Administration (FDA) considers non-THC based hemp products to be "food based" and, therefore, legal without a medical marijuana license. CBD Rich Hemp Oil is legal in all 50 states. And not any of the cases presented in this book is in violation of the United States Controlled Substances Act (US.CSA).

Table of Contents

ACKNOWLEDGEMENTS

"The Healer Within" began as a messenger with a message, powerful yet subtle; a synthesis of my research and discoveries that I gathered over the years, and still exploring and developing through my *Healer Within.*

This project would not have been possible without the contributions of two talented souls.

The research, translation, and literary efforts of **Stella Gimenez** kept me going during the most trying parts of this project. Without her, this would be an entirely different book.

Brian M. F. Burch, and his impressive editing skills, patiently transformed my years of collected research into the thought-provoking, life-changing book you now have in your hands. For his help, I am forever grateful.

And finally, I express my deepest gratitude *To the Stars*; to all those *Highest Beings* that "wanted" me to write these messages to you; to the inspirations I've received from these highest guides.

This book is for you, for whenever you are ready to hear these messages that are not from me, but from *"them"* to *"you"*.

<u>INTRODUCTION</u>

This book has been living with me for over thirty years. Each healing experience became a chapter, and each chapter a new learning process through the unquestionable cure provided by nature and our authentic mind-body connection.

I am so grateful for the ability to reach so many people through this book who I would have never met otherwise. Life is a such a miracle. To know that people across the world will learn to overcome physical and mental disorders from knowledge I'm able to teach in this book leaves me in awe.

I realized I am here to spread the word about a special natural healing process that has cured me and others over centuries and across the world.

I became interested in the healing of diseases years ago. My personal experiences, and those of loved ones, have heightened my awareness of these paths through a self-conscious healing process. They have opened my mind and made me be a strong believer in natural medicine.

I believed and experienced that both disease and healing are created by our own habits as a learning experience. Just as we created the disease, we can also heal it from within ourselves by changing our habits of belief and awareness.

While some scientific minds might find this very controversial, there are several well-known proofs, found all over the world, of people with severe physical and mental conditions, that have received "inexplicable" natural cures and remissions, leaving the "rational" science without any scientific explanation.

I also believe in the use of all kinds of natural healing methods as opposed to drugs. Pharmaceutical drugs have their place in emergencies, but they do not perform well for long term usage. Cancer is still considered a terminal disease, in most cases, and usually treated with life-draining chemotherapy, with a shockingly low success rate of only 3%! [i] Radiation treatments usually cause more harm than good. Many times the cancer is cured but the side effects often end up killing the patient themselves.

My experience with this is personal, with both of my parents and many friends dying from cancer "treatments."

During my expansive research on natural medicine, I practiced energy healing, meditation, and yoga in order to keep my Healer Within strong, able to heal myself, to prevent illness, and to naturally guide those I consult. Most of all, what I learned is that we can't separate our mindful consciousness from our mindful body. The two are bonded through a high level of communication, and through their dialogue we can continue learning and mastering our living laboratory.

Besides our mind-body connection, it is well proven that the healing properties of natural medicine including plants, herbs, their extracts, and homeopathic medicine, combined with a balanced diet and exercise, are capable of preventing illness and creating health.

So, I thank you, the reader, for this opportunity to share with you the knowledge I have acquired and make this world a healthier place, one person at a time.

William Pieper

2016

Section 1

Modern Medicine, Incorporated

With this book, I don't intend to denounce with the full names those physicians who practice fraudulent medicine and dramatically ruined the physical and financial well-being of their *"patients"* and families. It is already in the news that many *prominent cancer* doctors were forced under oath in court to admit that they wrongfully and *intentionally* diagnosed healthy people with cancer.

Rather, I intend to raise awareness about doctors who, protected under a title and a prestigious medical career specialization in cancer, are abusing the innocence of their patients by prescribing them very expensive and dangerous treatments. These patients and their families have later discovered their lives have been ruined and buried under mountains of debt.

Patients continue to fall into the hands of deceitful doctors who diagnose a so-called "incurable" disease they don't have, driven solely by greed. Building business, profits, or their egos have trumped the importance of their patients' health.

So many people have tried alternative medicine for cancer and received their cure. Did they really have it? Was it a combination of faith, healthy treatments, and prayers, or they might have been misdiagnosed?

"The art of healing comes from nature, not from the physician. Therefore, the physician must start from nature, with an open mind."
- Philipus Aureolus Paracelsus

The good news is that these fraudulent physicians are getting caught! The bad news is that we are unable to recognize when a doctor is truly helpful and trying to heal us, or giving us poison through, for instance, chemotherapy and radiation, simply to drive his profits.

The worldwide industry that has been created to *"cure"* cancer impedes the development of a reliable research to prevent and truly cure cancer. It's well known that international cancer funds invest a mere pittance of their funds toward cancer prevention when compared to the enormous amounts of money devoted to executive salaries and researching chemotherapy and radiation. If cancer were cured or prevented, the entire cancer industry would be out of business. The big money is cancer treatment, not prevention.

While it may come as a shock that a doctor could use a fake a diagnosis to become famous and/or a millionaire at the cost of his or her *patient*'s life, this awful crime not only happens in the cancer *"industry"*.

Many medical doctors around the world who promised to dedicate their career to the cure and well-being of their patients have become greedy, and unscrupulous physicians. They treat patients as *"clients"* and build their business on the trust of their patients. They have become physicians without a conscience.

When money is involved in the field of *"health"*, the life of a person can be destroyed under an irreparable harm when the doctor knows that the treatment they prescribed is *"medically unnecessary."* Several doctors have increased their incomes through the commissions they received according to the volume of patients they treat and continuing treating with specific medicaments.

Take the example of prostate cancer. Statistics said that 90% of doctors that prescribe cancer treatment for prostate, generate a commission from each treatment their patients receive.

While prostate cancer does not always turn out to be a deadly condition, about only 3% of men suffering from prostate cancer die, it is possible that the PSA test can create false-positive diagnoses and lead to biopsies and treatments that usually cause impotence and incontinence.

A study published by the New England Journal of Medicine revealed that a mammography has caused more damage than benefits to the women who have employed it over the past 30 years in attempt to fight breast cancer. The study says that mammography appears to have *created* 1.3 million cases of breast cancer in the U.S.! [ii]

75% of doctors refuse chemotherapy on themselves if diagnosed with cancer. [iii]

And while chemo only succeeds in beating cancer 3% of the time, chemo itself kills the patient 7.5% of the time! [iv] By doctors' own admission, chemo kills more than twice as often as it saves! This number – 7.5% – represents cases where it is indisputable that chemotherapy is the cause of death, but in reality, chemo probably kills much more often.

The cancer industry promises effective cures while promoting their patented, expensive, and poisoned chemicals, the risks or which far exceed any benefit, and they do it because it makes money. Unfortunately money, greed, and profits run the worldwide pharmaceutical industry. If the cancer is eradicated, so are their profits.

There is no governing force to protect us. Americans enjoy the delusion that the FDA is protecting us from harmful food and drugs, but the FDA is literally run by pharmaceutical and medical field executives.

Predator doctors are so common that it's quite possible you or a friend or family member have been a victim, but recognizing their uncompassionate and greedy behavior won't give us our health back, nor will it recoup the money and time we wasted in intoxicating treatments. The more we know about the corporate mentality of modern medicine, the more opportunity we will have to better understand our symptoms but the cause of them.

We are taught to believe that cancer happens on its own at random, that the way we live, think, feel, act, eat, and managing the massive waves of stress have nothing to do with it. Therefore, we may have no choice but to accept poisonous chemotherapy, burning radiation, and the possible mutilating surgery doctors will prescribe for us.

It may sound too late, but it is not. We must learn how we provoked our disease, and how we – and only we – can reverse it.

Even facing the devastating news, we have the enormous power to change the way we have been living, believing, reacting, eating, drinking, and other habits to improve our health.

Yes, there are doctors who, either intentionally or by ignorance, damage their patients with extremely dangerous treatments. Yes, there is a large industry ever increasing their wealth at the expense of the irreparable harm done by labeling a healthy person as "sick." Above all, it is in our hands, in the wisdom or our spirit and body-mind connection, where we can find the field for our own cure. There is a cure, and it comes from within ourselves by changing harmful habits and beliefs. The cure will truly heal us when we release negative emotions, resentful thoughts, anger, hatred, fear and despair.

"Every human being is the author of his own health or disease." -Swami Sivananda Saraswati

It takes commitment, tenacity, and follow through to change, to develop new patterns, to undo what is threatening our lives. We need to persevere with self-control to resist addictive behavior, and to give ourselves space, time, and love to learn everything we need to become even healthier than we were before our diagnosis. We must gather our courage when others demand we surrender to traditional medicine, despite the irreversible side-effects of their treatments. We are capable of taking charge of our own health and to change the habits and behaviors that have caused a disease.

As J.J. Goldwag suggested in his inspirational ideas about healing ourselves from within, we shouldn't give illness our attention by repeating the story of it over and over again. Instead, we need to focus our mind on all the positive areas of our life and we will see how often our sickness will receive *the message* and fade away.

It is crucial to be proactive about our healing goal, starting from within our mind-body connection, healing our emotions, and changing negative beliefs into positive behaviors. The results will be seen in our cured body. We are the extraordinary proof of how much loving ourselves and others provide us the unique healing process that goes beyond scientific comprehension. The more we focus only on positive thoughts and feelings, the better life we can achieve, ensuring the well-being of ourselves and everything and everyone around us.

We all know- but we often forget – that life is constantly changing, and every living being, including you and me, is included in this process. We must learn not to resist, but to go with the flow of life. We need to trust in the wise messages of our circumstances without allowing fear to influence our decisions. The *"comfort zone"* is a trap that will paralyze us into an uncomfortable state of illness. We must take responsibility for the health of our bodies, rather than entrusting that responsibility to strangers.

Every commercial for the newest and greatest medication paints such a beautiful picture of what life can be, yet comes with a ridiculously long list of *"possible dangerous side effects?"* This adverse secondary effects should give us the idea that we probably won't get healed but, instead, get worse. We may not be sick to begin with! We may find ourselves in exhausting tests and treatments at the expense of our health. We may lose our jobs. We will most certainly lose our money! Then, physical and emotionally ill, we will find ourselves in a hopeless and helpless state of being.

Let us commit, right now, to a plan to create the best lives for ourselves, no matter how young or mature we might be. While allowing ourselves to evolve toward a better quality of life, we will contribute to our constant healing process. The practice of building our full communication with our inner healer will become our most powerful medicine to overcome any illness we face on the road ahead.

Habits, right or wrong, are solidified through repetition. Avoiding the repetition of your unhealthy behaviors will be the first step to getting rid of them. We will clean our inner home while welcoming health, in all its forms, to be manifested within, and we will maintain these healthy habits for life.

Section 2

Achieving Optimum Health

The Spark

My awareness of the *Healer Within* comes from a place outside of me, from a time when I was still in space traveling in the sky. I have no memories from this time. Somehow, I know I didn't travel in a spaceship. I was merely an intelligent being without a body, centered within an infinite spark of light. Me as a "Self" was this spark of light.

Even though I have made my crucial adjustment to Earth and have made many mistakes, something wonderful and inexplicable keeps me connected to this time and the vast possibilities of space. I receive joyous whispers of who I am and where I came from in my ordinary life.

When I turned five, my granddad gave me a telescope as a birthday present. He told me secretly, *"Now you can see all those stars you love to reach when you fly on my shoulders. Now, you may see your home."* Then he softly stroked my head, and with a twinkle that started in his smile and made its way up to his eyes, he turned and walked away.

I have had vivid dreams that brought me to a healing place as well. In one distinct spiritual experience I envisioned I was somewhere in the Amazonian rainforest as a Medicine Man danced and chanted around me. I was gently spinning in the curling white smoke of burning *palo santo*. The aromatic smell woke my senses before I even opened my eyes. A very deep sense of wellbeing aroused within me, and I was able to maintain that feeling for several months.

I often fly in my dreams. In one unique and very vivid dream I soared into the beyond. It was this dream that revealed in my life the "presence" of the Divine Spark.

The sequences of flying dreams began, as usual, with me sprinting. From a central point on my forehead, I was able to channel the inspiration required to lift myself from the ground and started flying not higher than a two story building. Then, for the first and only time in my dreams, a powerful force pulled me up without my consent. I wasn't able to fight against this strong "determination," and, as I ascended, I gradually lost everything that could represent *"me"*. I was vividly conscious that I was losing my body, my personality, my ego. Nothing at all remained in "me" for someone to say: "Look, there goes our friend!". Then, I arrived at a realm of full, brilliant, amazing, infinite sparks of lights.

Unconditional love, compassion, peace, happiness, and well-being were simultaneously present as I had never experienced before. *I was one of those infinite sparks of light!* I remember saying to "myself": *Ah! I know who we all are. We all are one of these sparks of light. We still have unconscious memories of our Divine Source, and everything we do on earth is to regenerate this rewarding state of being within ourselves.* When I woke up I felt myself in a higher level of consciousness. It was three o'clock in the morning. The state of peace and unconditional love became intertwined with every aspect of my ordinary life.

Each of these experiences and dreams became a calling - a persistent reminder that compels me to unleash the power of my spark, and tells me that I know how to allow the healing process to flow through me. This knowledge keeps me enthralled with what is beyond, and I prefer not to dwell on small things or the past, but rather in terms of the stars.

At times I have wondered about this message, even looked in the mirror and said, "Me?!" But my dreams and healing experiences inspire me.

I am aware of how much harm we receive when we are disconnected from the natural conversation of the spirit, body and mind, and I have embarked on a search that has taught me to no longer be a fragmented person.

Divine Power

As soon as we are born, our ego, that dimness that always wants to own us and overshadow who we really are, constantly tries to move us away from our divine power. It makes us believe in doppelgangers, the unenlightened part of us that has us asking "Who am I?", telling us we can return to our magnificent, divine home through consumption, through beer, a party or movie. It tricks us into accepting our identity from the outside darkness, from our appearance, from superficial and cultural ideas we inherited along generations. But if we remember, we can quiet the ego and relearn that which we already know. We can connect again to our essences and open our hearts. We cannot do this by thinking and believing small, because our real selves are bigger than that. We can enhance our lives to a higher level only by thinking and believing in proportion with the stars. Only when we live through our mind-spirit-body connection, when we seek the purpose of our lives from and through the heart, will we experience the power of who we are, and who we are is far greater than who we think we are.

Somehow, unconsciously, we "remember" our true home, that realm that holds a constant creation of divine sparks. Therefore, everything we do on this planet is in search of that state of divine wellbeing, love, trust, forgiveness and compassion that we still deeply feel as a very silent trace of memory. The journey to get back to this place, however, is riddled with thorns.

The comforting force of our inner spark, the source of unconditional love that we all have within us, constantly is providing us with health, peace and happiness. It gives us the intuition that the act of defragmenting must come from within us, and that we have everything we need to nurture and heal ourselves and others.

Drugs' and Doctors' value and limitations

Even though, medications are necessary to help us go through serious medical conditions, we do not give our mindful connection the opportunity and the time to heal, before we take to pills and potions.

Doctors, nurses or surgeons do not heal us. It is our healthy mind-body connection that releases healthy and natural medicine from our *Healer Within.* Yes, we need a doctor to remove an infected appendix, but it is our innate body intelligence that makes us heal properly.

Our body has been divinely created to induce a powerful healing program in us. We should learn how to support ourselves and trust in our wisdom within.

Story: Stella & Diego

The miracles of life are ultimately expressions of something that begins deep within us. It all starts with our inner power being free from attachments and to shed the false beliefs that we have acquired culturally. When we go through this process, we become seeds of life's miracles for us and others. The story of my friend, Stella, and her elder son are a beautiful example.

From her childhood, Stella grew up intuitively listened to the fluent dialogue between her mind, her spirit and her body. Her oldest son, however, did not.

Diego grew up listening to his rational mind. He was a student of philosophy, history and social sciences. It was difficult for him to accept the powerful influence of the mind talking to the body. He did not believe that the spirit also takes part in that inner talk.

In 2001, Diego was diagnosed with a very aggressive carcinoma that attacks mostly young males. At the time, most of the people diagnosed with this cancer did not survive more than four months. The doctor spoke to Stella privately and said to her, "Please, do not tell your son, because we need him emotionally strong, but Diego likely has only four months left to live." Stella looked at the doctor of the hospital of Barcelona and said to him, "You do everything that you need to do, and we will do everything that we need to do."

Nobody told him, but Diego imagined that his life was in danger. He wanted to live, and he asked Stella for "alternative" help. They went together along the path of "dissolving" negative beliefs, of releasing labels, and of learning to live without attachments. Diego raised his mind-spirit-body connection through guided visualizations, prayers, yoga and meditations. He released all the toxins he had consumed in so many different ways and purified both his body and mind. He consciously gave up his fears, anxieties, manuals of "how to behave" and crippling beliefs. He replaced these negative emotions with faith, joy and hope. In this way, he removed his body from a devastating disease and elevated it into a state of peace and relaxation, allowing the Healer Within to conduct its work.

In 2015, Diego's doctors told him that he is the only one of their patients to have been cured. They now take his case to all the conferences where they present treatments against this aggressive type of cancer. They say that science has no explanation for the healing that Diego has received. They call him the miracle of the cancer hospital of Barcelona.

Like Diego, you, too, can shed the habits that hinder your health. Together, we will learn to awaken our own Healer Within.

What Is Health?

Health is not limited to the body. In order to experience optimum health, your body, mind, and spirit must all be healthy. They are all connected. Each influence, and is influenced by, each of the others.

If the body becomes sick, the mind and spirit are then sickened by the body. If, however, your body is generally healthy, but your mind is sick, your body won't stay healthy for long, as the negative patterns of the mind will soon manifest in the body.

Your environment influences your mind, body, and spirit. Mind, body, and spirit all influence each other, often communicating with emotion, and all ultimately affect your vibrations. Vibrations then dictate your health.

So, where do we start? At what step do we have control to stop harmful patterns and habits and reestablish optimum health?

We can have influence on all of these areas of our lives. On the following pages, you will find many of the tools you need to optimize health in your body, mind, and spirit, tips on developing mind-body-spirit communication, as well as some additional environmental improvements.

I warn you, you cannot focus on just one of these areas, and you cannot let any of these categories slip, or the Healer Within will not be fully free. Mind, body, and spirit are inseparable. Any imbalance can, and probably will – cause significant change to spread through your entire body. Optimum health is about total balance, with the Healer Within flowing throughout you, energizing and inspiring every aspect of your being.

Mind-body history
The idea that a person's well-being is dependent on a healthy body-mind-spirit interaction is not new.

For thousands of years great minds from the East to the West have been teaching the importance of awakening and maintaining our mind-body connection to keep us living a healthy life. The founding fathers of Western medicine such as Galen, Hippocrates and even Plato claimed that our emotions played a key role in causing our illnesses. The etymology of *"health"* even comes from the old English *hælþ,* meaning *"wholeness, being whole".*

Homeostasis
Ultimately, what we are after is homeostasis. This is a maintained internal balance. When you have built up healthy habits in mind, body, soul, environment, emotion, and vibrations, this state of homeostasis makes it next to impossible for

sickness to occur at all. As soon as one area becomes sick, whether it's a virus, bacteria, thought, broken bone, pulled muscle, depression, or whatever, the sickness is rejected by the overall healthy being, and optimum health is reinstated. Homeostasis is maintained by overall healthy habits, and sickness in all its forms is literally repelled by it.

Positively influencing from the body

Our body, the biological part of ourselves, needs to be nourished with healthy food, activities, and most of all, with a positive mind-body dialogue.

We are capable of healing ourselves from severe and terminal illnesses through positive attitudes and by improving our belief that our *Healer Within* is taking care of us, physically and emotionally.

Consumption Habits

In the course of our daily lives we may consume toxic food, alcoholic beverages or drugs. This distorts our mind and body connection, causing all kinds of negative emotions. Meanwhile, we produce a vicious cycle of increasing intoxication. The adverse reactions are anger, fear, resentment, and suicidal behavior, among other dangers.

When we decrease our craving for unhealthy food, drinks, and other toxic consumables, we are able to better tune ourselves to the messages that our bodies are sending to us. Many times we eat without being hungry, or drink without being thirsty. We are so focused on "appealing" foods and drinks that, in spite of knowing they are not good for us, we still follow the instincts of our cultural behavior from past generations. When we turn off our appetite for self-damage, we are able to intuitively perceive what our healthy (or unhealthy) body is trying to tell us.

Often when we think we are hungry, we are only dehydrated. Our body may crave food only as a source of hydration, since most of the water our bodies need comes from food. If you find yourself hungry, try drinking a glass of water first.

If we fill our bodies with sustenance containing high vibrations, like natural fruits and vegetables, we merge with and become these high vibrations. Likewise, if we consume low vibrational foods, such as highly processed and unhealthy junk foods, we merge with and become these low vibrations. What we eat is what we become.

Smiling

I was walking along a busy city street one day, when I happened upon an old homeless man. As soon as I passed by him, he extended his right hand and, with a genuine smile on his face, he asked me: *"A smile, please..."* His candor, gentleness, and his smile requesting for "a smile", improved my mood immediately. He lit up my day. He made me smile to him, to me, and to my difficulties. I gave him a smile of gratitude and some money as well.

I always knew the smile's ability to improve moods and health, but it was with that brief interaction when I got my Eureka moment. Since then, I never leave a smile behind.

Neuroscientists have recently learned what wise and spiritual people have already known for centuries: The power of a smile! *Every time we smile, we send good instructions to our brain to release a full state of well-being through our mind-body connection.*

Smiling is a perfect example of our body's influence over our health. You part your lips and your cheeks rise, and neural messaging is activated, releasing positive, health supporting chemicals you're your body.

Smiling stimulates the release of neuropeptides – tiny molecules that produce neuronal connection – such as dopamine, endorphins and serotonin that are responsible for reducing stress. Endorphins are well known as a natural pain reliever without any of the adverse side effects provided by synthetic medicine. Serotonin acts as a mood lifter/anti-depressant.

Smiles are free, they don't need a doctor's prescription to improve your emotional state, and they don't provoke any negative side effects in your mind-body connection. When we smile we are manifesting gratitude, blessings, friendship, confidence, a loving approach others, but it also helps in lowering our blood pressure, our heart rate, and stress levels.

Our smiles project light from our inner wisdom. They open doors and alleviate suffering. They are magnificent rainbows in the storm. They build up hopes, an attitude that can demolish the hardest circumstances we may be facing now and then in our human life.

Enjoy increased attractiveness by smiling, because prefer to be close to people who have a relaxed face than to those whose faces look sad, tense, worry or irritated. A relaxed face creates fewer wrinkles, extended youth, and harmonious feelings inside and outside.

We can all experience the benefits of smiling. These benefits don't take longer to be manifested. They are simultaneous with the power of a smile.

Exercise
This doesn't have to be vigorous three hour daily gym visits. Just avoid lethargy. Our bodies are meant to move.

In 2008-2009, the average American watched four hours and forty-nine minutes of television *per day!* [c] The average American also works eight hours a day.

With such sedentary habits, it is no wonder disease is on the rise.

Get up, go for a walk or run. Put on your favorite music and dance! Start a game of kick-ball in the yard with your neighbors! Let them laugh at you from their couches!

Many have been pressured by their culture to sit in an uncomfortable chair and stare at a computer screen for eight or more hours in the day. If this is what your job requires, take the initiative to take breaks to get up, stretch, and walk around for a few minutes. Your body will thank you, and, although you spend less time working, studies show you actually get more done! [d]

Relax
Relaxation will contribute to the rewiring of our brain in a healthy way. With so much pressure to achieve and push ourselves to succeed, sometimes what we really need is to take some time and relax.

Lethargy is certainly not a healthy lifestyle, but neither is constant pressure on acquiring more things, and achieving more goals.

What is optimal for your well-being is balance. Set goals, have drive and passion, but don't forget to relax sometimes.

Positively Influencing from the mind

STORY: 75 Year old Stroke Survivor

I met once in a park, a man seventy-five years "young", walking his dog. We began to chat. Even though what he said didn't surprise me, while listening to his true story a pleasant feeling showered over me. During his youth, he was a Catholic priest in Mexico. Later he realized that he didn't belong to that world of what he called "fake faith". He started living the life of a free man without being attached to any religious belief. He was as happy and unhappy as anyone in the world.

He denied the existence of a God and a Divine Source above us. After several years of being a single man he married and had a daughter who became his purpose in life.

Then tragedy struck in the form of a severe stroke. He was no longer able to speak or move properly. Doctors gave him no hope for recovery. He looked at his daughter and he realized he needed to do something. But what?

Then he got inspired. He remembered his time as a priest, and started focusing on a healing prayer he once knew. Although he couldn't speak, he was able to manage an inner healing speech through his mind. Every day, many times, he prayed. He didn't allow any negative feeling to discourage his goal. He just focused on his prayer. A year later he started moving the disabled parts of his body. Then he learned to walk again with the help of a cane, and later, without the cane. He practiced, slowly and patiently, his ability to speak, and he was able to speak normally again.

As he told me his story, I never would have guessed that this man had such a sever stroke only two years prior. His eyes were peaceful and his smile very soothing.

I left him with his dog and the happy feeling of his achievement. I know that when we awake our Healer Within, we can experience such a high state of health, which brings us to a more positive attitude. These experiences inspire us. It pleased me to met a person who was able to transform his life by empowering a mindful awareness in the here and now. It is never too late to heal ourselves through a balanced mind-body connection. Let us develop faith that the Healer Within will release our natural resources to cure ourselves.

The Power of the Mind over the Body

The combination of feelings and rational thoughts first takes place in our mind, and from there goes to the body. What our minds processes can and will affect our bodies, body and mind in a constant dialogue when we are awake and asleep. When our brain rewires itself through positive thoughts and feelings, we are rewarded with a healthy attitude that will be reflected in a better emotional and physical condition.

When we think about some particular food we like, and it is time to eat, our mouth will release saliva. This and other examples of thoughts triggering body responses occur because our subconscious mind doesn't realize the difference between a real experience and an imaginary experience. This example gives us enough evidence of how thoughts can provoke a chemical reaction that parallels its physical manifestation.

Say a bear jumps out of your closet. Of course you will be scared, and probably should be. You panic, and your brain will release chemicals like adrenaline and cortisol that tighten your muscles and increase stress. This is perfectly natural.

Now, let's say you have a fear that there is a bear in your closet. What happens? Your brain releases chemicals like adrenaline and cortisol that tighten your muscles and increase stress! Your body cannot tell the difference between the thought and the real threat. Your body gets the same message either way.

Many people live their lives in fear, and their bodies stay in a constant state of stress, wreaking havoc on their overall health. How do we fix this? We must not identify with our thoughts. We observe our thoughts, and release the ones that are not helpful to us.

Fearing bear in your closet causes only harm. It does not help us. We must trust in our intuition that if, one day, a bear does jump out of our closet, we will act appropriately when the time comes.

A bear in the closet may seem ridiculous and irrational, but it is no more irrational that the majority of fears people carry with them through their entire lives.

Fearing real threats right in front of you, like a bear, is natural and healthy. Fearing scenarios you imagine in your mind causes only unnecessary stress for your body, because it can't tell the difference. Imaginary scenarios, restricted only to the mind, are the cause of the vast majority of fear in the world. The unnecessary stress this causes to our bodies leads to a laundry list of illnesses, and can be stopped simply with awareness.

A continuous release of cortisol, a steroid hormone, in response to daily stress may harm our immune system, lead to weight gain, cause blood sugar imbalance and diabetes, gastrointestinal problems, heart problems, fertility problems, and so on.

It is important to learn where our power lies. Thoughts come and go all day long. Our power lies in the ability to let go of these thoughts, to recognize these thoughts as imaginary and unhelpful, and go on about our daily lives.

While imaginary fears affect our bodies negatively, imaginary pleasures can affect our bodies positively. Anytime we allow ourselves to feel a very vivid rewarding experience, our brain sends signals to our body. Just a particular thought, filled with pleasant emotions of previous physical satisfaction, triggers instant emotional and physical responses.

Power of beliefs

Our minds have power to affect our reality. What we think is what we feel. Empowering beliefs can result in a better and healthier life than circumstances can.

Science has demonstrated how our physical body is in direct communication with thoughts and feelings. Our beliefs produce a strong effect on how we interact with our physical, mental and emotional bodies.

For example, researchers at Caltech and Stanford have proven that wine connoisseurs prefer the taste of the $45 bottle of wine over the $5 bottle, even though they're drinking the same stuff! Simply by seeing a fancy label, they actually *experience* a tastier wine. They believed the wine was better, and it created their reality. [a]

People pay three times as much for Starbucks, even though McDonald's coffee beat Starbucks in a blind taste test. [b] Beliefs trump reality time and again.

A lady told me once that when she wants to have a glass of red wine, and there is not any around, she drinks a glass of water recreating in her mind the taste, the texture, the smell, and the pleasure having wine.

And while the common retort is to say that empowering beliefs may deny reality, remember that we have no idea what reality is. Everything is an illusion. We experience the world through the filters of our limited senses. Beliefs are all we have, so we might as well choose the most empowering beliefs to live by.

Placebos
Sometimes placebos are given to produce a healing process only because our mind

believes that we are "receiving healing medicine". These beliefs encourage our mind-body connection to release the healing process that flows naturally when we keep our faith high and without expectations.

Discovered during WWII when morphine was scarce, Dr Henry Beecher needed to operate on a wounded soldier, but had no pain killers. His nurse injected the patient, and the patient became relaxed and without pain. Yet, he was only injected with saline, and the placebo effect was discovered. [e]

Placebos, "medicine" with absolutely no medicinal qualities, can have positive effects on depression, pain, sleep disorders, digestion issues, and menopause.

Placebos can lead to very real chemical changes in the brain and body. A patient takes a placebo, and their brain releases opioids for pain relief, or dopamine for better movement and neurotransmission.

If a person with an illness takes a placebo, which is essentially just a sugar pill, and the illness goes away, the undeniable conclusion is that it was not the pill that healed him, but the Healer Within.

We can learn from the placebo effect to have faith in our Healer Within. The belief that the Healer Within is working to fight disease and keep us healthy is a necessary step in achieving optimum health, and often, as with placebos, the only thing that is missing.

Healthy attitude

A healthy attitude can rescue us from the most traumatic experiences in life.

Dr. Viktor Frankl, and other survivors from a concentration camp, are vivid proof of how we can create a better state of mind, in spite of the harmful experiences we may be receiving from outside circumstances. The technique they used, either consciously or unconsciously, was not to absorb the fear, the pain, and all the disturbing emotions from their environment. Instead, they chose to focus on the here and now; breathing in, breathing out, practicing a compassionate attitude towards those things they were not able to change.

Dr. Frankl and the other survivors increased the influence of their compassion instead of developing fury and hatred. They have chosen not to judge, but to witness their emotions from a neutral point, to remain in a balanced state of mind that decreases stress, to transcend horror without being damaged within themselves.

Positive Thinking

Do not underestimate the power of positive thinking. Keeping a positive, optimistic mindset does wonders for your overall health.

We already know the power our minds have over our bodies, so commit now to remain positive all day every day, and reap the benefits of higher energy, less stress, and smooth flowing body-mind communication.

It is easy to recognize the negative thoughts, not only because of the emotional effect it will have on you, but you will also feel its effects on your body. When you notice a negative thought in your head, immediately choose to replace it with a more positive one.

"I'm so tired," can be replaced with, "I have unlimited energy." "I'll never get out of debt," can be replaced with, "There are unlimited resources at my fingertips, and Mother Earth always provides what I need." Even if it feels silly at first, once you recognize the increased health and quality of life this habit brings shortly after enacting it, you'll never go back!

Learning and Growing

Learning and growing applies to every aspect of your being. It can help your body to learn to ride a bike or swing a golf club. It can help your mind to learn calculus or a foreign language. It can help your spirit to learn the deepest truths of reality through meditation.

The old adage "When you're through learning, you're through," is quite accurate. When one ceases to grow and evolve and experience, he becomes stagnant, and this will most certainly lead to sickness.

Maintaining mind, body, and spirit is to grow your mind, body, and spirit. Learn new skills, and never stop challenging yourself to become greater than your current earth-state. (I specify earth-state because ultimately we are all perfect beings.) You may not be aware of what amazing things you're capable of.

Create

We are all born with divine creativity. It is a part of who we are. Many of us s ay "I'm just not a creative person," and let that part of ourselves wither away. Of course, we are all creative. Those that can't seem to create only have the ego blocking their creativity.

We are all creators, every day in our lives, whether we realize it or not. Begin to embrace it, express your creativity, and you will revive parts of your being necessary for complete health.

Attachment vs Detachment

Unconsciously, and culturally, we tend to plug ourselves in or attach to all manners of things. Some of our attachments may include dreams, things, success, failure, love, hate, desires, me, you, him, her, and our constant race toward a fulfilling life.

It is a fact of life that change is constant. Resistance to change is attachment, and is the cause of all misery. Everything,

44

including you, is in perpetual transformation. When we fail to release people, events, situations, or anything else from our pasts, we become misaligned with reality, skewing our mind-body-spirit connection. The body is always present, so if our mind is not, the discrepancy damages the mind-body connection, and disease ensues.

The Healer within tells us to stay detached from everything and everyone. Do not confuse detachment with lack of love. It simply means that to avoid the causes of our physical distress, we should unplug from the expectations and attachments that bring us only frustration, sadness or feelings of unworthiness. It means that the only dialogue we should maintain is the one that pairs with our mind-body connection, the one that keep us healthy, the one that may contribute to the healing process of others and with nature. Through detachment, we set ourselves and others free from dependency.

Attachment stems from a belief that you are not enough as you are. In fact, you have everything you will ever need, and you always will. It is scary to let go of your attachments. Trust in your spirit to provide you everything that you think your attachments provide, and practice letting go.

Frequencies and Vibrations

Alexander Graham Bell speech about frequencies

"Suppose you have the power to make an iron rod vibrate with any desired frequency in a dark room. At first, when vibrating slowly, its movement will be indicated only by one sense: that of touch. As soon as the vibrations increase, a low sound will emanate from it and it will appeal to two senses. At about 32,000 vibrations to the second the sound will be loud and shrill, but at 40,000 vibrations it will be silent and the movements of the rod will not be perceived by touch. Its movements will be perceived by no ordinary human sense. From this point up to about 1-1.5 million vibrations, we have no sense that can appreciate any effect of the intervening vibrations. After that stage is reached movement is indicated first by the sense of temperature, and then, when the rod becomes red-hot, by the sense

of sight. At 3 million vibrations it sheds violet light. Above that it sheds ultra-violet rays and other invisible radiation, some of which can be perceived by instruments and employed by us. Now it has occurred to me that there must be a great deal to be learned about the effect of those vibrations in the great gap where the ordinary human senses are unable to hear, see, or feel the movement. The power to send wireless messages by ether vibrations lies in that gap. But the gap is so great that it seems there must be much more. We must make machines practically to supply new senses as the wireless instruments do. Can it be said when you think of that great gap, that there are not many forms of vibrations that make up results as wonderful as, or even more wonderful than the wireless waves? It seems to me that in this gap lie the vibrations that we have assumed to be given off by our brains and nerve cells when we think, but then again they may be higher up in the scale beyond the vibrations that produce the ultra-violet rays." – Alexander Graham Bell [f]

Intro to Frequency

Many of us may not be looking to discover the "secrets of the universe," but if we are trying to understand what is manifesting in our lives, it is beneficial to know that everything is energy. Thoughts and emotions actively participate in a dialogue that takes place on a vibrational level.

Energy is vibrating at different frequencies all throughout the universe. Everything that is seen and unseen, whether perceived by our senses or not - feelings, thoughts, dreams, physical bodies, objects, subtle forces and tangible ones - are fields of vibrational energy.

The vibrational field is everywhere. It vibrates both at our individual level, and in the whole universe. Vibrations create reactions in our emotions as our perceptions are stimulated by vibratory input. Within our vibrational field, there is a constant dialogue that communicates energy in all its infinite forms.

When our mind is processing a thought, be it rational or emotional one, we release it as a frequency that vibrates, creating something somewhere and in someone. If the frequency of our thoughts is negative, it affects others negatively, and they produce negative frequencies which then affect you negatively, and the cycle continues.

The vibration of positive thoughts, however, combined with positive feelings, will expand a healing wave on us, our environment, and our relationships. We become vibrational healers of ourselves, of everything, of everybody. We can even heal the past by traveling through healing thought back to the moment the wound was created.

Emotions of anger may have their roots in deep fears. Later, they can become resentment. Led by our ego, anger and resentment create a damaging poison that returns to us in the form of deathly illness and mental disease. We make ourselves and others sick. We also create, without being completely aware, a negative frequency in the places we inhabit. We start attracting dark forces that feed themselves through our fears, anger, hatred, resentment, and unforgivable feelings. They grow within us, fed by the vicious cycle of negative thoughts until we are consumed by the dark field of helplessness.

"The molecular arrangement of the physical body is a complex network of interwoven energy fields. The energetic network, which represents the physical/cellular framework, is organized and nourished by "subtle" dynamic systems that coordinate the life-force within the body. There is a hierarchy of subtle energetic systems that coordinate electrophysiologic and hormonal function as well as a cellular structure within the physical body.

It is primarily from these subtle levels that health and illness originate... these subtle energies influence cellular patterns of growth in both positive and negative directions." -Richard Gerber M.D., Vibrational Medicine

We are different beings with various levels of physical, mental, emotional and spiritual energy.

Each energy possesses a vibrational frequency, which then combine to create the vibration of our being, and also the environment in which we live, our home, work, and relationships with others. Much of what we experience can be understood as dialogue between vibrations.

Like attracts like. Low-frequency vibration attracts other low-frequency vibrations, and high attracts high. According to how we vibrate in our subtle energy levels, we can draw positive or negative results into our lives.

When we observe that our lives have been affected negatively, we realize it occurred because the frequency of our energy levels declined. We have allowed – no, we have *invited* negative emotions and fears into our presence.

We have the power to attract all things we desire with the collaboration of our emotional and rational thought, flowing together in the same level of commitment. Therefore, nothing is a consequence of luck. We rebuke what others call luck. The power of our intention is magnificent, and we have great power if we use it properly. It is our great ally that fulfills our lives - even when life is uncertain.

Shapes & Chi

We are constantly bombarded by the vibrations of our environment, relationships, memories from the past, worries about the future, and decisions in the present. Whether we are aware or not, our vibratory system is regularly and harmfully affecting us with damaging electromagnetic frequencies, from every house appliance, television set, computers, electrical poles, cell phones, microwave and so many outside influences.

The shape of an object delivers a message that may not be instantly understood by our rational mind, but instead, it becomes a subtle communication within the field where emotions affect our perceptions.

Over millennia, Chinese masters have practiced a technique called Feng Shui, which is used to facilitate the flow of Ch'i energy. They observe how shapes, of any kind, can affect the harmony of a place and how it is transferred to impact our emotions.

When we see a form that may be interpreted as harmful or pleasant, our whole body reacts. These reactions, sometimes, are filtered by our rational mind that suppresses the authentic message coming from the intelligence of our emotional body.

Feng Shui masters teach that we should avoid a shape that transmits *"sha"*, evil energy or an energy able to harm us.

I experienced this energy in action one day when a friend of mine, who loves to play with evil masks to perform "something funny," put his evil mask on to show me what he was planning to wear for Halloween. What followed amazed me.

My friend has a German Shepherd dog that he got when the puppy was no more than forty days. His name is Fredo. Since he came to my friend's home, Fredo slept with him and followed him everywhere he went. The moment my friend put on his horrifying mask, the dog ran away, almost crying and with his body in a posture closer to the floor.

The natural intelligence of the dog made him received the negative frequency emitted from the shape of the mask.

Vibrational Healing History
Vibrational Healing is not a new idea, and has, in fact, been around since our early stages of evolution. Formulas for Vibrational Healing have been found in

ancient Egypt, where the use of sounds and color combined with herbs and harmonious smells contributed to the well-being of the ill person.

The Chinese have developed the idea of the meridians, lines of energy across the body, which reveal the relationship between a point and centers of "chi" that are affected by illness. People from India, as well as other far East and millennial cultures, like Tibet, Nepal, Mongolia, have used, and still use today, the powerful vibration of healing chants through the repetition of particular " mantras", dances, movements and herbs.

Western countries have adopted ancient techniques as a healthy and natural vibrational healing system, noninvasive and without side effects. Vibrational medicine can be found through: healing sounds, guided imagery, harmonious smells and beautiful scented natural lotions, massage, bath, prayers, meditation, relaxation, homeopathy, healing herbs. Any of these vibrational methods can deliver healthy and long-term results. It also creates an evolutionary transformation in those who practice, and in those who receive the benefits of vibrational medicine of any kind.

Water

Masaru Emoto was a Japanese author, researcher, and entrepreneur who believed that human consciousness has an effect on the molecular structure of water. Water is able to react with positive thoughts and words as well as negative intentions. It can also be cleansed through prayer and positive visualization.

Emoto demonstrated that emotional "energies" and "vibrations" can transform the physical structure of water. He believed that shapes, words, pictures, and sounds have a powerful influence in developing good or bad quality of water. According to his results, frozen water that was exposed to positive emotions, speech, and thoughts, visually formed harmonious crystals. Conversely, negative intention manifested hideous forms.

In the documentary Water: The Great Mystery, which I highly recommend, the molecular *structure* of water is shown to be a significant factor in our body's reaction to it. All water is made up of two parts hydrogen and one part oxygen, but how these water molecules are structured makes a major difference. Positive thoughts and vibrations, such as those discovered by Masaru Emoto, create molecular structures of water that are healthier for us with higher energies. Water that has never experienced human interaction, such as those found by scientists in 2009 on the Roraima plateaus of Venezuela, has the most advanced molecular structure found to date, and has healing properties due solely to its energetic purity. To contrast, common municipal water practices include starting with polluted water, often mixed with human waste, saturating it with chlorine, and pumping it through rusty pipes to your faucet. As expected, this municipal water has very low energy structures, and contributes to the general unhealthiness of humanity. [h]

Thoughts & Vibrations affect DNA

While exploring vibrational behavior of DNA, Russian biophysicist and molecular biologist Pjotr Garjajev discovered a powerful healing force in which DNA can be influenced and reprogrammed by words and "frequencies."

The emission and reception of certain levels of "frequencies" can explain mental phenomena such as intuition, remote communication, clairvoyance, telepathy, prayers that perform healing along the distance, self-help affirmation techniques, self-healing highest lights emitted by spiritual masters, and the positive or negative influence coming from the intention of the mind.

A whole new kind of healing has been developed, influencing and reprogramming our DNA and its genetic inheritance.

"Only 10% of our DNA is being used for building proteins. It is this subset of DNA that is of interest to western researchers and is being examined and categorized. The other 90% is considered "junk DNA."☐ The Russian researchers, however, convinced that nature was not dumb, joined linguists and geneticists in a venture to explore those 90% of "junk DNA."☐ Their results, findings, and conclusions are simply revolutionary! According to them, our DNA is not only responsible for the construction of our body but also serves as data storage and in communication. The Russian linguists found that the genetic code, especially in the apparently useless 90%, follows the same rules as all our human languages. To this

end, they compared the rules of syntax (the way in which words are put together to form phrases and sentences), semantics (the study of meaning in language forms) and the basic rules of grammar. They found that the alkalines of our DNA follow a regular grammar and do have set rules just like our languages. So human languages did not appear coincidentally but are a reflection of our genetic DNA." - Pjotr Garjajev [j]

Through repeating positive affirmations and being under the relaxing influence of guided imagery or hypnosis, we can produce powerful effects on every living being including humans, animals, plants, and the whole planet.

Pjotr Garjajev and his team have developed devices that can positively influence our cells through modulated radio and light frequencies to repair genetic defects.

Influencing Frequency
High vibratory frequencies are filled with:

- The mindful relationship between mind-body-emotion

that achieves harmonious well-being in ourselves, others, and the environment.

- Awareness that everything we think and feel is becoming part of ourselves and is our reality.
- A communion of mind-body-emotional flow that will keep us in a healthy state of neutrality.
- Appreciation of beauty in all it forms.
- Consciousness of what we consume.
- An attitude of abundance, but a life without excess.
- A peaceful state of being that can be achieved through meditation.
- Dance meditation.
- Walking meditation.
- Free movement meditation.
- Still meditation.

- Sound meditation.

- Expressing gratitude.

- Compassionate behavior.

Vibrational healing works better through the power of intention. It is crucial to be truly aware of what energies we are send or receive, and how it might affect those around us. Willingness to explore the different layers of our physical and subtle bodies will enable us to receive profound waves of healing messages into our vibrational field. These waves will harmoniously balance our whole self by creating a peaceful sense of well-being.

In her infinite wisdom, Mother Nature communicates within and between the interactive and universal vibrational field. Her powerful essence manifests the perfect balance between beauty and health. She also has the wisdom to reestablish balance when it has been lost.

Plants, crystals, pleasant aromas, beautiful views, shapes, and harmonious sounds can heal energies that are out of balance in our energy fields.

Vibrational remedies release their powerful healing messages on our subtle levels. Our mind craves only facts and rationality, keeping us in a vicious circle of illnesses if other factors are ignored. Vibrations can pierce through the barriers of our rational mind. The more we permit our senses to interact with harmonious vibrations, be it sounds, smells, textures, shapes, colors, positive thoughts, or feelings, the higher our level of energy will rise, and the healthier we become.

"Emotions have unique vibrations just like colors and physical objects do. These emotional vibrations also go from higher/faster to lower/slower. When you are laughing and having fun, your body's vibrations are lighter (higher and faster). When you are tired and sick your vibrations are heavier (slower and lower). You know how when you are in love, you feel "energized", "high", like you're "walking on a cloud?" That's because your emotions are literally adding voltage and power, lightening your body. And when you're negative and depressed, you feel sluggish,

"feeling low," "heavy". "I'm down today."
Your emotional vibrations are giving your
body a slower, lower vibration. This is not
speaking metaphorically. This is
scientifically measurable." -Molecules of
Emotion by Dr. Candace Pert and HMI

How to increase the level of our Emotional Frequency

Our healing purpose doesn't have to, and
often won't satisfy our ego or the appetite
of our instincts. Raising the level of our
emotional frequency is to bring us mental,
emotional, and physical well-being. This
attitude will strengthen our connection to a
higher vibrational field of consciousness.

Mastering our intention to evolve into a
higher frequency is a process that needs our
constant commitment, and it only happens
in the present moment, when we are fully
aware. High frequency is a lifestyle to be
maintained, not an achievement.

Each of us has the power to choose high
frequency over low frequency. This
exercise in integrity not only helps us
continually evolve into higher realms, but
also inspires others to follow suit.

When we practice being in a high-frequency level, we will experience miracles. It may seem like a fairy tale but it is true. Everything we intentionally manifest will let us achieve our goals. We will experience a state known as "the flow".

Positive intentions

Applying vibration and language can become a powerful influence in the healing of our cells.

What science is proving and experiencing today, has been practiced by esoteric and spiritual masters for centuries. Our body can be programmable by sounds, words, and thoughts. We just need to use the positive intention of harmonious vibrations to lead our cells into their healthy and natural balance.

Anybody can do this. The only vital requirements are to do this with an authentic positive intention without the interference of any negative thought, without ego, and from a healthy environment. The better the atmosphere, the better the healing effect.

Many cultures in history knew of the healing power of words and thoughts. Mayans, Native Americans, African tribes, and many others have been known to hold healing festivities with healing mantras, chants, and music. The healing effects of these sounds and intentions were relied upon for the health of their people.

Maintaining "flow" and good vibrations
How to attain a neutral state of flow:

- Lower all distracting noises that come from conspiring thoughts - they will regularly travel from the past to the future in an eternal trip to nowhere.
- Let go of the "ego" and its army of negative emotions.
- Practice mindfulness to remain in the "present moment".
- Elevate Low-Frequency Emotions into High-Frequency Emotions.
- Nurture High-Frequency Emotions in spite of any threatening circumstances that may appear in our way, either from within or outside of us.

High-Frequency Emotions do not have any "ego" that feeds us with selfish and aggressive behaviors. Emotions that nurture high frequencies include:

- Love – Compassion
- Enthusiasm – Trust – Faith
- Courage – Gratitude
- Joy – Acceptance – Inspirations
- Hope – Optimism – Care
- Unselfishness – Understanding

Low-Frequency Emotions are driven by "ego," and they behave reactively to anything that contradicts them. Low Frequencies are manifested by:

- Pessimism – Selfishness
- Irritation – Impatience
- Frustration – Criticism
- Disappointment – Anger
- Aggression – Blame
- Discrimination
- Revenge – Worries
- Unworthiness – Arrogance
- Hatred – Jealousy – Fear
- Depression

Because illness and disease are developed by imbalanced conditions, a vibrational healing treatment can be implemented simply by putting forth conscious effort towards increasing your frequencies and balancing the vibrations in our physical and subtle bodies.

Anytime we are under a deep influence of distress, it provokes imbalances in our cells, organs, and our energetic body, greatly weakening our immune system.

To live a healthy life, we must maintain a high vibrational level in our physical and subtle bodies. When our energy flows in a healthy rhythm, it nourishes our feelings, our healthy mental activity, all our senses, and the power of our self-defense against any disease.

When our frequencies become unbalanced, our vibratory mind- body communication is clouded, or even blocked. We become more susceptible to negative invaders, and our health declines.

Our physical and subtle bodies have their particular vibrations.

How we feel emotionally has been created by a unique vibration. Colors, smells, light, darkness, unhealthy food, healthy food, thoughts, desires, sounds, touch - everything has its special way of vibrating.

Emotions

Emotions

When we believe a situation is hopeless, think no one will listen to us, or accept that we cannot rise above a haunting memory, we cultivate a serious combination of negative emotions in our life:

- Fear
- Anxiety
- Anger
- Resentment
- Criticism
- Sadness
- Hopelessness
- Ego
- Control
- Attachment

These negative emotions fuel diseases like cancer, draining away our strength. Conversely, positive emotions promote youth, energy, healing and happiness. Making them a natural part of our lives means overcoming the ego, letting go of fear and embracing forgiveness.

Ego

Most of the time, we believe that "we" react, rationally or irrationally, to things that try to harm us, but this belief is not true. It is our *ego*, not our true heart, that reacts.

The ego responds aggressively in this way because it doesn't like to be seen as "less than", a "fool", "ignorant" or "useless". But our real self sees through the lies and knows its own worth.

The spark understands the truth of who we are, and it doesn't view us according to the distortions or expectations of anyone else. Thus, when we rise above the ego and listen to our divine power, we can behave motivated by compassion instead of offense, trust instead of fear. We can prevent potentially negative outcomes and manifest a relaxed and detached attitude, inspiring in others a better model of an evolutionary behavior.

If we cannot heed our inner spark, our ego takes control, and fear becomes our unrelenting ruler. We fear the idea of ceasing to exist, physically or from the mind of those who are so important to our lives.

We fear separation, abandonment, rejection, humiliation, embarrassment and being deemed unworthy. We fear the idea of losing any valuable part of our body, of being immobilized, restricted and controlled by circumstances beyond our control and will. We develop anxiety about the possibility of external sources like contagious illness, insects, criminals, natural disasters, war, or *dark forces from the unknown* continuously threatening our lives. All these fears increase our anxiety, and anxiety increases the negative emotional energy that interferes with our natural healing process. We doubt our powerful inner self. We lose trust in ourselves to handle life's challenges. We resort to jealousy, paranoia, anger and blame. We disconnect the flow of energy that heals us through the healthy dialogue between our mind-body connection.

The problem of the ego and fear-based behavior is bad enough on its own, but it is even worse considering that we all are born with an extraordinary ability to "pre-create" our future throughout our imagination and even to place ourselves physically into that imaginary scenario. This ability can be an amazing tool toward success if we use it the right way and imagine positive events. Unfortunately, we tend to use it to preconceive an imminent threat, instantly an uncontrollable anxiety and overwhelming distress.

Anxiety's effect on the body

In the 2012 New York Times article, *"Searching the Brain for the Roots of Fear"*, neuroscientist Joseph Ledoux (*) explains how fear and the ability to imagine often lead us to unnecessary suffering.

"We actually know a tremendous amount about what goes on in the brain when stimuli present during danger become memory triggers for the danger. To make a complicated story very simple (though not inaccurate) a region in the brain called the amygdala connects the two events, forming an unconscious memory of the association. When the neutral stimulus (the rock or the sound of an airplane) later occurs, it automatically activates the amygdala like

the original danger did, eliciting fear, and also triggers worry — anxiety. The automatic nature of the activation process reflects the fact that the amygdala does its work outside of conscious awareness. We respond to danger, then only· afterward realize danger is present.

Every animal (including insects and worms, as well as animals more like us) is born with the ability to detect and respond to certain kinds of danger, and to learn about things associated with danger. In short, the capacity to fear (in the sense of detecting and responding to danger) is pretty universal among animals. But anxiety — an experience of uncertainty — is a different matter. It depends on the ability to anticipate, a capacity that is also present in some other animals, but that is especially well developed in humans. We can project ourselves into the future like no other creature.

While anxiety is defined by uncertainty, human anxiety is greatly amplified by our ability to imagine the future, and our place in it, even a future that is physically impossible. With imagination we can ruminate over that yet to be experienced, possibly impossible scenario. We use this creative capacity to great advantage when we envision how to make our lives better, but we can just as easily put it to work in less productive ways — worrying excessively about the outcome of things. Some concern about outcomes is essential to success in meeting life's challenges and opportunities. But at some point, most of us probably worry more than we need to. This raises the questions: How much fear and worry is too much? How do we know when we have skipped the line from normal fear and anxiety to a disorder?

Fear and anxiety are in the brain because they helped our ancestors and theirs cope with life's challenges. But when these states interfere with our ability to survive and thrive, one has an anxiety disorder. These include phobias, panic disorder, post-traumatic stress syndrome, generalized anxiety disorder, among other conditions. While fear plays a key role in some anxiety disorders (phobia, post-traumatic stress), it takes a back seat in others (generalized anxiety).

Pathological fear and anxiety are due to alterations of the brain systems that *normally control fear and anxiety (structures such as the amygdala). A tremendous amount has been learned about the normal system from studies of other animals. This gives us a good shot at understanding the pathological forms, and developing ways to treat and maybe even prevent them. Indeed, recent research in animal models are giving us new clues about how to treat problems of fear and anxiety in humans, both pharmacologically and behaviorally, and helping us figure out how we can pull people back once they've crossed the blurry line."*- Joseph Ledoux

Ledoux is not alone in seeing the connection between emotion and the creation or cure of disease. In his book, *"The Instinct to Heal: Curing Depression, Anxiety and Stress Without Drugs and Without Talk Therapy,"* French neuroscientist Servan-Scheiber synthesizes the biology of our behaviors in the following way:

"Inside the brain there is an emotional brain, a real brain inside another brain. There, a different architecture arises with a different cellular organization, and with biochemical properties different from our

cerebral neocortex; that is to say, from the most evolved part of the brain where one gives place to language, consciousness, thinking. In fact, the emotional brain often works independently from our cerebral neocortex.

Language and cognition have limited influence: they cannot command our emotions so easily.

The emotional brain, controls everything what it governs psychological well-being and a large part of the corporal physiology as the functioning of our heart, blood pressure, hormones, digestive system and up to the immune system."- Servan-Scheiber

Under Servan-Scheiber's concepts, unresolved emotional conflicts may interfere with our natural aptitude to heal ourselves. Forgiveness, we learn, is a very important part of the healing process. By asking for or giving forgiveness, we dethrone the *King Ego,* which manifests its power over others through abusive and aggressive behavior. We unveil fear to be the destructive enemy of light that it is, bring with it anger, resentment, criticism and other negative feelings that prevent good health.

Emotional Health and Presence

Let us be led by our emotions, while a mindful attitude flows through a constant state of the present moment, to nourish our inner wisdom within our receptive awareness.

Allow us to be led by emotion through a conscious activity. It can be very healing to be guided by the emotional flow of our energy without obstructing or denying it.

While allowing ourselves to trust, we will become the flow and the observer. It will take us to moments of transcendence, of learning from a continuous evolution, that we would not have come to had we not trusted the wisdom that *"Let it go"* can offer us.

Our emotions are energies seeking to express themselves through our consciousness. Criticize them, delete them, hide them, and they will manifest themselves through signals that appear in our body. If we continue to deny emotions, over time they will be expressed with symptoms and even terminal diseases.

Guided Imagery
Guided Imagery is a powerful technique that can help us to awaken the *Healer Within*. We produce images in our mind which can generates emotions. This is a tool we can use to put our bodies into optimum healing states.

Several studies have proven the physiological impact of relaxation in inhibiting the release of the hormone cortisol, which enhances our body's response in moments of stress. A continuing release of cortisol, responding to daily stress, may harm our immune system, which is needed to be in balance to successfully fight against autoimmune diseases and cancer.

Oncologist O. Carl Simonton developed a particular type of guided imagery designed exclusively for use by cancer patients, used successfully in combination with conventional cancer treatment, reducing the use of more chemotherapy and radiation.

Through *Guided Imagery*, patients with cancer can realize a profound healing relaxation. Some of these visualizations involve mentally picturing how the body's immune response fights and destroys cancer cells. One of the exercises is to imagine the cells of our immune system as Pac-Men gobbling up and making the cancer cells completely disappear.

Guided Imagery exercises such as the Simonton Method motivate patients to interact consciously with the disease instead of being in a passive role. It allows patients to reach a state of health and confidence and develop an improved outlook on the quality of their life.

Guided Imagery is a superb example of how our brains and bodies cooperate, creating a powerful healing experience through the use of imagination. It helps our emotions and thoughts work together to achieve the same goal of optimum health. *Guided Imagery* can generate a powerful experience as if it could be happening from outside stimuli. The brain can't tell the difference!

Processing Emotions

Do we run through life or is it life that runs through us? Does time fly without us being aware of it? Many of us tend to participate within the rhythm of life without awareness about how to consciously dance in it. Some other times we *"wake up"* through a reaction against something that bothers us. Or we make mistakes – which is natural – and we chase them with sorrows, regrets, or anger – which is harmful.

Emotions can't be manipulated. That is worth repeating: *Emotions cannot be manipulated.* Emotions are the natural process of mind communicating with body. They are meant to be received, accepted, and released.

We have the ability to *influence* our emotions through habits and thoughts. However, once an emotion is present, you must accept it.

Our natural state is in pleasant emotions, and it is our responsibility to release the bad ones mindfully and harmoniously, receive the message, and release it to make room for the god ones.

Our emotions circulate throughout our mind-body communication. These emotions transport their *"voice"* through connections that actively participate within our endocrine system, gastrointestinal system, our immune system, and the brain. This intelligent, emotional communication freely flows, delivering messages along our mind-body consciousness.

We don't need to dominate or repress our emotions. All emotions, even the unpleasant ones like anger and fear, possess deep and divine intelligence. Emotions are our bodies' way of communicating very important messages with us. We need to develop the wisdom to improve our mind-body connection to receive their messages and let them flow freely.

When we try to ignore, repress, or deny our inner communication, our body will manifest symptoms, phobias, and diseases. This constant and interactive voice that flows naturally within our mind-body connection must be heard through our awareness in order to experience optimum health.

Some people believe that by releasing their emotions, regardless of how much they may harm others, it is the right thing to do. Releasing negative emotions, to free them without thinking, or realizing that they are creating harmful consequences for others, will provoke the poison arrow to return to us without being aware of it. It won't bring any solution, but an increasing amount of damage to ourselves and others.

Freeing emotions; dark ones, happy ones, joyful ones, can be easily done by a harmonious mind-body movement. Stress has been part of our evolution, as a powerful skill to defend ourselves from threatening circumstances. We need to release stress by moving our bodies, otherwise stress will overwhelm us with poisonous remnants like cortisol. That is why 'movement', and most of all harmonious conscious movement, like dancing, will free harmful emotions and create in us a healthy flow of healing energy. Repressed anger, sadness, hatred should be liberated by going for a mindful walk, dancing, singing, exercise, an authentic prayer, or mindful meditation

Vibrations & Emotions

The chemicals released when feeling positive emotions create a constant flow of healing energy.

Negative emotions manifest themselves through discordant waves. They are dissonant, and flow in broken frequencies.

We don't need to suppress our negative emotions, neither to release them toward others, ourselves, or our environment. We need to practice how to tolerate the energies of grief, fear, anguish, sadness or despair, while allowing them release through our mind-body connection. During the natural process, we will learn from the positive wisdom they have brought into our lives.

A mindful awareness immerses us in the tolerant process of allowing negative energy to flow, bringing us the experience of receiving messages coming from our emotions.

Find your Point of Balance

Spending just a little time for oneself can be the most powerful healing process one will ever receive.

By practicing the mental power of our self-healing vibrational energy, we can discover Point of Balance. The Point of Balance is a state of harmony, the source from where our whole self can create calmness, peace, and the miracle of mental and physical healing.

Imagine a healing place that is being harmfully shaken by an earthquake. It doesn't matter how many machines and doctors practicing the best medicine with the latest technologies there are, once the shaking begins, it becomes out of balance and the healing procedure can't occur. The same happens to us when life shakes us with difficult circumstances. We break down under conscious and unconscious distress. Anytime we keep ourselves within the Point of Balance; we will experience how much wisdom we have to heal ourselves.

Our body and mind, together and in balance, have all the power necessary to maintain health in the flow of perfect harmony. When we live a stressful life we are in the earthquake moment, shaking and destroying all our possibilities to prevent illness, and blocking the healing connection.

Alternatively, when we are in an integrated mind-body connection, we will quickly reach a balanced state of well-being. From this neutral point, we will become fearless and confident. We can cultivate the seeds that will unfold a subtle yet powerful release of healing forces that will free us from mental and physical illness. Yes, we can. We can transform ourselves from a weak and powerless state to become our highest healers.

There are so many examples of people who created miracles in their lives by spending time on their Point of Balance, letting go of all the causes of stress that were the primary causes of their illness. Science is still researching how these seemingly impossible cures have happened.

Some medical doctors dodge the word "miracle" by variations of the following line: "under the law of our medical treatments we cannot explain these cures." Yet, the patients *are* cured. It is totally possible. We don't need to be the "selected ones from heaven" to experience the healing responses of our body-mind connection when we allow the healing process to happen within our peaceful and balanced state of being.

Let's try to focus on breathing in and breathing out. Releasing tensions, and freeing all kinds of thoughts and sensations that disturb this state. Witnessing our thoughts without trying to suppress them, we let them flow and go.

It is not easy because we are not accustomed to quiet the storm of our thoughts and emotions. This triggers fears, distress, anxiety, and despair. We can train ourselves to be in the here and now, to be where our body is, neither in the past nor future.

Benefits of Meditation
For decades neuroscientists have believed that as our brain ages it affects the quality of our lives, and we can't do anything about it. Through the latest research, it has been proven that our brain has neuroplasticity. MRI scans of meditating patients have shown extraordinary improvements in brain function compared to the scans of patients who are not meditating.

Maintaining our mental health in this way is an important part of mind-body communication, and, therefore, overall health.

Benefits we can achieve through meditation:

- Relaxes our mind and body
- Creates calm state for sleeping
- Helps us improve our immunological system
- Releases our distress
- Promotes tolerance
- Develops positive feelings and behaviors
- Normalizes our blood pressure
- Balances our endocrine system
- Activates our mind-body connections
- Puts us in a state of awareness
- Enhances intuition

Mindful Meditation

Accept your difficulties. This is a wise first step to prepare for a meditation.

It is difficult for many of us to achieve a healing state of relaxation while waves of thoughts overwhelm us with worries, fears, and anxiety. At this point, we may not be aware of how much tension is taking over our bodies.

We may find excuses to avoid a regular practice of meditation because we think we can't control our thoughts. We don't need to, but instead we should allow them to come, acknowledge them, and release them without passing judgment on them.

Mindful meditation isn't about getting rid of your thoughts, although quieting your mind is a nice effect you will enjoy. Rather, mindful meditation is about mindfulness, about being aware of your thoughts, your body's reaction to them, and how they are affecting you. It is your reaction to the thoughts that cause illness much more so than the thoughts themselves.

Meditation should have no goal in mind. There is nothing to acquire that you don't already have. All you're going to do is observe. You may notice things going on in your mind, body, emotions, or receive important messages directly from your inner spark. Or, you may notice nothing, and be easily distracted through the process, or become uncomfortable, all of which are natural and acceptable. The meditation still has its value, regardless of what happens during the process.

Taking a few minutes focusing your mind on breathing in and breathing out will be enough to start training yourself in the quest to develop the consciousness of our Healer Within.

Each time thoughts and feelings appear, observe them without evaluation as if watching the clouds passing by until the sky becomes clear. We are neutral witnesses, letting go of worries. Notice these thoughts and emotions occur within you, but are not you. You are not these thoughts, but merely observing them. Do not become attached.

We don't need to go anywhere to reach the healing state of well-being. Mindful meditation can be done anywhere.

We are not forcing anything. The Healer Within does not take orders. Rather, what we're doing is *allowing* the Healer Within to do what it does naturally when it's not shackled by stress and distraction. Our inner wisdom holds all the medicine in the Universe to spread healing energy all over the different layers of our being.

Start with five minutes, twice a day, and with practice you can extend these sessions by a few minutes each day. Twenty minutes of meditation daily is enough to see significant benefits in your stress levels, mind-body connection, and health. If you are the ambitious type, hours of meditation daily can lead to serious spiritual enlightenment, and even transition to higher plains.

Soon, you will find yourself more mindful in every waking moment of the day. Through practicing mindful behavior, we are able to tolerate negative emotions, minimizing the emotional damage. When we learn how to tolerate unpleasant emotional energy, we will understand and learn from them. We can act instead of react. Then, we can control our words and actions instead of being controlled by them. We can transform ourselves into a continuing evolutionary being.

Section 2 summary

The habits that lead to good health are simple, but so rare in today's culture. As we as a people forget these habits, our health, and the health of the world, declines, as it has been steadily for decades. Yet, there is good news in this, and that is that you have the power to reclaim your right to optimum health simply by adopting the healthy habits listed in this section.

Exercise, relax, eat right, and smile to keep your body healthy. Maintain a positive mindset, learn, and adopt positive beliefs to keep your mind healthy. Meditate to keep your spirit healthy. Cherish, understand, and process your emotions to keep your mind-body-spirit connection flowing. Do all of these things, and you will be healthier than you ever have before, and disease will be a thing of the past.

These habits are so easy, yet they are equally easy to drop or stray from. Constant pushing from marketing magicians, family, friends, work, culture, government, and an endless amount of other sources do their absolute best to distract you from achieving and maintaining optimum health and keeping the highest vibrations. Therefore, the final thing needed to achieve optimum health not yet mentioned in this section is *will power* to create and keep these habits in your life.

There is another tool that Mother Earth provides for us, both as help to maintain these habits, and as a supplemental supporting habit, which is so effective it has received its own Section, which follows.

Section 3

CBD: The Miracle Supplement

What is CBD?

Cannabidiol (or CBD) has so many benefits it's no wonder the medical industry wants it to remain a controlled substance. This natural supplement single-handedly has the potential to wipe a large portion of the medical industry's profits off the map.

Cannabidiol is one of over a hundred chemical compounds found in Hemp. Along with numerous real and direct health benefits of cannabidiol, hemp provides mental & mind-body-spirit benefits, dietary benefits, textile production benefits, and even renewable energy potential. The financial damage this plant can do to many of the world's largest corporations leaves little wonder why there is so much misinformation spread about hemp.

In this section, you will learn the vast array of benefits provided by hemp, particularly CBD, and how you can – and why you should – incorporate CBD into your mind-body health regimen you designed in Section 2.

Definitions

Hemp, Pot, Weed, CBD, THC, marijuana, cannabis, cannabinoid... it's all the same thing, right?

Far from it. We have decades of misinformation to thank for the confusion, and you'll learn why soon. For now, let's clear things up.

Cannabis

Cannabis is a Genus of plants which, with hops (a brewer's favorite), is in the Cannabaceae family. Humans, or Homo Sapiens, are in the Homo genus of the Hominid family.

Marijuana

Cannabis Sativa, a particular species of Cannabis, well known for its high THC content. The term was coined by Hearst-owned newspapers in the 1930's during a campaign to ban hemp production.

Hemp
Hemp is the plant.   There are different strains of hemp, including cannabis.   All cannabis is hemp, but not all hemp is cannabis.

Cannabinoid
The chemical compounds found in hemp. THC and CBD are both cannabinoids.

Cannabidiol
One of over one hundred chemical compounds found in hemp. Cannabidiol is the main focus of this section do to its remarkable health qualities.

CBD
CBD is simply the abbreviation for Cannabidiol.

THC
Tetrahydrocannabinol, or THC, is the most widely known chemical compound found in hemp, especially marijuana.   THC is the compound that produces a physiological reaction.   In other words, THC is why marijuana gets people high.

Hemp oil
The oil extracted from the hemp plant.

CBD oil
A concentrated hemp oil that has very strong levels of CBD and typically very low or non-existent levels of THC.

History of hemp
Hemp is been known, used, and even revered throughout recorded history and across the world. Rightly so, as you will agree as we discover the near-miraculous properties of the plant.

Neolithic history
There is overwhelming archeological evidence that the Japanese cultivated hemp for clothing, paper, and food as far back as 10,000 B.C. E. To this day, many Kimono designs feature the character for hemp.

In China, hemp fiber imprints were found on Yangshao pottery dating back to 4800 B. C. E. As China matured as a nation, hemp's use was expanded to produce clothing, shoes, ropes, building material, and paper.

In 2013, archeologists digging near the Kunar River in Pakistan discovered a site they believe to be over 2500 years old. The artifacts showed hemp being used both as a medicinal treatment and in ceremonial rituals.

Hemp in the U.S.

In fifteenth century Europe, hemp was widely used to produce high-quality textiles and garments to be sold in town. It should come as no surprise, then, that even the ropes used on the ships of Christopher Columbus were made of hemp.

It was Spanish, in fact, who brought hemp to the Western Hemisphere and began cultivating it in Chile around 1545. By May 1607, hemp had made its way north as far as Virginia, where it was observed being grown by natives. Samuel Argall, English adventurer and sea captain, observed wild hemp growing along the banks of the Potomac in 1613.

Our founding fathers were well versed in farming hemp. George Washington encouraged hemp growth in America, and set the example by not only growing it himself, but smoking it for its medicinal qualities. His diary mentions harvesting twenty-seven bushels of hemp in 1765. He said to his gardener at Mount Vernon, "Make the most of the Indian hemp seed, and sow it everywhere!" Other supporters of hemp included Thomas Jefferson, James Madison, James Monroe, and Andrew Jackson. Even the Declaration of Independence and the Constitution were both written on hemp paper.

Hemp use was a large factor in the U.S. presidential Election of 1880, when Harrison ran against Garfield. Harrison's posters encouraged voters to "Protect American corn, hemp, rice, and fruit!"

If hemp has been so admired historically from 10,000 B. C. E. up through the 19th century, why do we find ourselves in these modern times with hemp prohibition in the United States? In fact, the U.S. is the only country in the world with a ban on growing industrial hemp!

"Why use up the forests which were centuries in the making and the mines which required ages to lay down, if we can get the equivalent of forest and mineral products in the annual growth of the hemp fields?" – Henry Ford

The Marijuana Tax Act of 1937 imposed a tax on anyone dealing commercially with cannabis, hemp, or marijuana. It is widely suspected the law was pushed through by businessmen like the DuPont family.

The DuPonts had a new material, polyester, that they wanted to sell. Their major competition was – you guessed it – hemp clothing.

In common U.S. Political form, the Du Pont Corporation hired lobbyists and greased the right wheels in campaign "contributions" (read "bribes"). DuPont's chief financial backer Andrew Mellon, Secretary of the Treasury in the Hoover administration, appointed Harry J Anslinger to head the Federal Bureau of Narcotics and Dangerous Drugs. William Randolph Hearst, owner of a chain of newspapers, began publishing enhanced stories of marijuana crazed criminals wreaking havoc across the country. It was these newspapers that coined the term and renamed cannabis "marijuana", and labeled it, "the killer weed from Mexico." Harry J Anslinger then testified before Congress that "Marijuana is the most violence causing drug in the history of mankind."

With such influence, the Marijuana Tax Act of 1937 was passed, despite the avid opposition of the American Medical Association! The AMA thought that hemp products would replace half of the painkillers on the market. From 1850 to 1937, hemp was the prime medicine for over 100 diseases in the U.S. pharmacopoeia. The official statement on the Act by Dr. James Woodard, legislative council of the AMA, included, "We cannot understand yet... why this bill should have been prepared in secret for two years without any intimation, even to the profession that it was being prepared... The American Medical Association knows of no evidence that marijuana is a dangerous drug." He also discouraged marijuana prohibition as it would deny America of its substantial medical uses.

The AMA eventually changed their official opinion of hemp to match that of Anslinger's. Of course, this was after years of encouragement of Anslinger, who prosecuted over 3000 doctors for writing illegal prescriptions.

The results of the Act were massive. 116 million pounds of hemp seed were used solely for paint and varnish. After 1937, most of that business went to chemicals produced by DuPont.

The Act laid the groundwork for the Controlled Subsatances Act, which categorized marijuana as among the most dangerous drugs, thus officially making marijuana illegal.

If you read section 1, this corporatization of medical treatment is no shock. The Marijuana Tax Act of 1937 is but one example of corporate greed trumping our health. [1]

Despite the Act, the U.S. government encouraged the growth of hemp to supply the troops in WWII with uniforms, canvas, and rope, having lost Japan as its major source for hemp imports. The government produced "Hemp For Victory", a short 1942 film, promoting hemp as the crop that will win the war.

Since then, corporate profits have remained the priority of U.S. lawmakers. Of course, marijuana and hemp have been prohibited, but also, the violators of the ban are prosecuted like violent criminals. As of 2014, half of inmates in federal prison were serving their time for drug offenses, and 47% of state prisons. [2] Not surprisingly, the most powerful opponents of any bill legalizing marijuana are always the corporations that run prisons. Yes, prisons are privately owned and managed.

25% of people on probation, and 32% of those on parole, had a drug charge as their most serious offense. [2]

The FDA has made it illegal to claim that anything other than a drug can cure a disease. CBD is a natural compound, and therefore cannot be patented like a drug. For these reasons, we may never see the day when CBD is prescribed by doctors.

Clearly, the legalization of hemp would cause large and powerful corporations to lose out on massive profits. Indeed, the very livelihood of many corporations relies heavily on keeping hemp off the market as viable competition to their products. Since these large corporations are the major contributors to modern politicians' campaigns, it is no wonder why the ban on hemp is so cherished by those in power.

Yet, the world is awakening. Truth is taking root, and little by little, progress is being made in reestablishing hemp as a major resource in the U.S. Enlightenment is beginning, however slowly, to overpower corporate greed. Legal hemp product imports have increased from $1.4 million in 2000 to $11.5 million in 2011. The pressure of the informed citizens, due largely to the free sharing of information over the internet, is beginning to match the influence of the corporations and their deep wallets. A citizen's vote is more valuable than corporate cash. In fact, any corporate cash received by a politician is invested into getting more votes.

Currently, the legal stances of hemp in the U.S. on a federal level, and each state, are evolving too fast to discuss. Whatever I write here would be outdated by the time it is published. Instead, visit my webpage at CBDenergetics.com to get the most current information on hemp legalization available.

The Many Uses of Hemp

Why are corporations so afraid of hemp? Let's explore the endless uses of hemp, and why hemp should be the preferred alternative to many of our modern, everyday products.

Most of the products you will read about are products of hemp that has been bred over decades to have very little to no THC. Of course, other strains have been bred to *increase* the THC content – and lower the CBD content – for the pleasure of those seeking a good high, but hemp carries with it far more gifts to the world than that.

It is important to know that hemp is significantly easier to grow than most of its alternatives, including corn, soy, and cotton, and certainly easier to attain and replenish than crude oil. Hemp requires no herbicide, and is in fact a herbicide in its own right! Minimal pesticides are required, as hemp is naturally pest-resistant. And hemp actually replenishes the soil it grows in, eliminating the need to rotate the crops of its alternatives. The benefits of growing hemp add to the efficiency of its already superior products!

Textiles

In 1941, Henry Ford built a Model T out of hemp, flax, and linen, the impact strength of which was ten times greater than steel. Note that this was four years after the heavy tax on Marijuana was jammed through Congress.

Yes, hemp can be used to make various products. Just like Crude oil makes everything from roads, tires, toys, and plastics, hemp can be used to produce fabric, rope, paper, hemp-crete (a concrete alternative), and even oil!

Hemp paper is stronger than wood based paper, and cheaper to produce. While wood paper requires bleach to whiten, hemp paper is whitened by simple hydrogen peroxide. Hemp paper is acid-free, so it won't turn yellow and brittle. And while wood paper can be recycled a maximum of three times, hemp paper is recyclable up to seven times.

Clothing made from hemp fabrics prove to be better insulators than comparable cotton products, with many benefits to boot. Hemp keeps you warmer in the winter and cooler in the summer. Cotton production demands massive amounts of water and pesticides, making hemp clothing much better for the environment. It takes three acres of cotton to produce the same amount of fabric as one single acre of hemp. Plus, hemp cloth is more comfortable on the skin, and lasts longer than cotton cloth.

Building products from carpeting to insulation, and from fiberboard to stucco, can be made by hemp in a more efficient, cost-effective, and environmentally friendly way. Pest free, mold free, rot proof, and fire resistant, hemp building products last up to five hundred years, and are all recyclable.

Led by visionary Henry Ford, hordes of car manufacturers, from Audi to Volvo, are beginning to use hemp in their composite panels for improved safety ratings. Both the Lotus Eco Elise and Mercedes C-Class contain hemp.

Hemp plastic is organic and made from hemp, a renewable source, and is fully biodegradable. Conventional plastic is made from crude oil, a non-renewable source, and harmful chemicals, and its production releases pollutants into our environment. Worse, still, plastic is non-biodegradable, and will remain in our landfills for millennia.

If being more environmentally friendly to its competition isn't enough, hemp will actually counteract the negative effects of its dirtier counterparts. Hemp can be used to clear impurities out of wastewater such as sewage, phosphorus, and chemicals. Through the process of phytoremediation (don't worry, there's not a test), hemp is also being used to clear radioisotopes from the environment in Chernobyl.

Fuel and oil

Hemp bioethanol and biodiesel is more environmentally friendly than fuels produced with corn, palm oil, soy, and sugar beet, and with less harm done to the soil. Hemp also grows more quickly than its competitors.

Biodiesel and bioethanol produce far less pollution than is crude replacement, and is far more renewable. Its exhaust smells like hemp, not gasoline. It contains no sulfur.

Biodiesel is the only alternative fuel that runs in any conventional, unmodified diesel engine. It is also safe to handle, biodegradable, ten times less toxic than table salt, and a high flashpoint of 300 degrees Fahrenheit (compared to petroleum diesel at 125 F). [4]

Hemp biodiesel can actually *extend* the life of diesel engines since it is more lubricating than petroleum diesel.

All these benefits come with matched efficiency. It is only a matter of time until Hemp takes over as our world's energy source.

Food
Food products from hemp can include seeds, milk, oils/butters, and cereals. Whichever form of hemp you consume, its health benefits are endless.

Hemp is a superfood in and of itself. A better protein source than meat, eggs, cheese and milk, hemp is rich in fiber, vitamins, enzymes, antioxidants, and Omega 3 fats. Maintain a diet rich in hemp, and maintain a healthy mind-body connection.

Raw hemp contributes to weight-loss, increased energy, lower blood pressure, lower cholesterol, improved circulation, boosted immunity, and a speedy recovery from disease or injury.

Hemp milk in particular is a great alternative to bovine milk. With fewer calories, low fat, vitamins, minerals, Omega 3 fatty acids, and no sugar, hemp milk does not spoil quickly, needs no refrigeration, and creates far less pollution than the modern cattle camps.

The Miracle of CBD

It is clear why energy, food, and manufacturing corporations fear the legalization of hemp, yet even this pales in comparison to the threats hemp poses to our modern pharmaceutical and medical infrastructure. In no small part to the ban on hemp, scientists have only scratched the surface of the benefits of hemp's chemical compounds, but CBD has already taken a leading role in these studies. Here's what we know so far...

Anti-inflammatory

CBD is a proven anti-inflammatory. Inflammation occurs at the slightest upset of mind-body imbalance, and leads to a host of other sicknesses and diseases. The Endocannabinoids have a remarkable effect on your body's inflammation by blocking glycine receptors. In other words, if something is slightly wrong with your mind-body balance, CBD will prevent excessive inflammation and keep you as balanced as possible.

While inflammation is the body's natural attempt to heal itself, our modern lifestyles, diets, and environments – or sometimes genetic predisposition – cause excessive and chronic inflammation, which leads to chronic pain, which leads to cancer, arthritis, asthma, tuberculosis, hay fever, Crohn's disease, irritable bowel syndrome, hepatitis, periodontitis, and heart disease, to name a few. [8] [9]

Inflammation is good and healthy for cuts and bruises, but the damage our bodies endure from our damaging lifestyles also causes inflammation, and our mind-body health spirals out of control. Hence, CBD will stop this process in its tracks.

Of course, a healthy lifestyle is necessary to long-term health and happiness, but CBD stops inflammation, allowing your body to more quickly achieve homeostasis.

Pain relief

CBD is a godsend for those suffering from chronic back pain, and doubly so because CBD is all natural and has no side effects. Some brave doctors are prescribing CBD as a moderately strong analgesic – a pain reliever – particularly for cancer-related pain and neuropathic pain. [10]

Perhaps the greatest pain relief CBD can provide is for the neuropathic pain caused by chemotherapy. However, studies show that regular CBD consumption over time will lead to lesser pain sensitivity of all types. [11]

Considering that every prescription and over-the-counter pain relief drug includes synthetic chemicals constructed in a lab and a long list of side-effects, CBD is worth considering as a natural alternative.

Arthritis relief

Studies show vast improvements in arthritis patients after regular doses of CBD. Along with Cancer treatment, arthritis is at the forefront of CBD medical studies. A controlled study at the British Royal National Hospital in 2006 had patients take regular cannabinoids over a five week period, resulting in significantly less pain and inflammation. The study also shows evidence of slowing the development of arthritis. [12]

Arthritis is essentially joint pain caused by years of chronic inflammation. CBD, as we already know, is a miraculous anti-inflammatory and pain reliever. This makes CBD an ideal supplement to both treat and prevent arthritis symptoms.

Cancer/tumor treatment and prevention

CBD is used somewhat commonly to treat side-effects of cancer treatment caused by chemotherapy and radiation treatments, such as nausea, loss of appetite, pain, and difficulty sleeping, but there is a wide array of evidence that CBD can actually treat and prevent cancer itself!

The California Pacific Medical center has been researching cannabinoids for over twenty years. They have discovered that

CBD has the ability to "turn off" the DNA that causes breast cancer, brain cancer, prostate cancer, and other cancers to metastasize. [13]

Another study shows cannabinoids inhibits the spread of cancer cells in lung cancer patients. [14]

In other studies, cannabinoids are shown to interfere and prevent tumors from forming by essentially starving them of the body's resources, which is bad for the tumor, but good for you and your body! [15]

As of 2016, the cancer treatment and prevention properties of CBD are already very promising, yet we have only scratched the surface in this area.

Anti-seizure and epilepsy treatment
In the years following Colorado's legalization of marijuana, families with epileptic children flocked to Colorado. Why? CBD is an all-natural, side effect free, non-psychoactive treatment for seizures.

It is an unfortunate fact that 30% of epileptic patients are entirely resistant to all modern medical treatments for the disease. For many of these drug-resistant epileptics,

Cannabinoids are the only treatments that work in reducing seizures. That these compounds have ever been banned is the real crime!

One study comparing common medical epilepsy treatment options versus CBD shows that CBD is equally effective as carbamazepine and chlordiazepoxide, and even more effective than phenytoin, trimethadione, and ethosuximide. Other cannabinoids, such as CBN and THC are also effective at treating epilepsy, but not as effective as CBD. The study also suggests that even greater results can be had when CBD is combined with some of the pharmaceuticals. [16]

A study in 1981 had epileptic patients combine CBD with their anti-convulsant drugs, and half of them became completely seizure free. 75% of the remaining half showed improvements. [18]

Another study in 1978 found that 200mg/kg doses of cannabis resin was 100% effective in stopping seizures! [17]

In an eerie twist, these anti-epileptic cannabinoid studies seemed to stop around

1982, which is suspicious considering the incredible results achieved in these studies. However, cannabinoids are making their comeback, and their medical benefits can no longer be hidden.

The Endocannabinoid System

The Endocannabinoid System, or ECS, is made up of a network of receptors primarily in the brain and nervous system, but also organs and tissues. The name may look familiar because it is named after the plant that led to its discovery. Before the effects of cannabinoids were measured within the body, scientists had no idea that this network in all of our bodies even existed. It's as if our bodies are made for cannabinoids.

All humans, vertebrates, and also sea squirts and nematodes have an endocannabinoid system. The cannabinoid receptors are embedded in cell membranes. When stimulated by cannabinoids, a plethora of physiologic processes take place, such as the ones discussed in this chapter. [19]

The cannabinoids react with the ECS receptors to create endocannabinoids –

chemicals made by our bodies – which bring all the benefits discussed herein. The endocannabinoids have a local effect and a short term influence on the body. [19]

"A functional cannabinoid system is essential for health," says Dustin Sulak, DO. He goes on to recommend regular CBD intake in small, daily doses to encourage our natural healing systems. [19]

Neuro-degenerative disease treatment and prevention

Studies have shown high iron content in the brain contributing to Alzeimer's and Parkinson's development. Luckily, CBD is an anti-oxidant, and has been shown to rebalance abnormally high iron levels in the brain, and regulate other chemical imbalances to boot. [20] Even a single dose of CBD was shown time and again to recover lost memories rats suffered due to high iron levels. [20]

CBD reduces neuroinflammation, the main cause of neurodegeneration. One particularly impressive study has shown CBD to actually *cure* mice with Alzheimer's disease, completely restoring their memory back to normal levels! [23]

CBD has been shown to improve the quality of life of Parkinson's disease patients. [21] Other studies indicate that CBD provides "significant, though temporary relieve from symptoms associated with... Parkinson's disease."[22]
I urge you all to check out http://www.parkinsonsrecovery.com/cbd to see an amazing 3 minute video showing the impact CBD has on one man suffering from Parkinson's. It is nothing short of miraculous.

Anti-psychotic

A research team at the University of Cologne in Germany showed CBD to have an equal success rate in treating schizophrenia as the anti-psychotic pharmaceutical amisulpride, except that CBD has absolutely zero side effects compared to amisulpride's laundry list of side effects. CBD also beat out amisulpride on the "negative symptoms" of schizophrenia, such as social withdrawal, reduced pleasure, and lack of motivation, although it is unknown if CBD helps to rid the patients of these symptoms, or simply causes fewer side effects to begin with. [24]

Anti-anxiety

CBD is shown to reduce anxiety in patients with different kinds of anxiety disorders. Social Anxiety Disorder affects 12% of Americans in their lifetime! The studies in this area are few, but CBD has massive potential to help those with SAD. [25]

Substance abuse relief

Cannabinoids are being used to curb methamphetamine addictions, [26] and is shown to actually *reverse* alcohol induced brain damage! [27] This is another example of CBD's anti-neurodegeneration principles.

Diabetes treatment and prevention

Type 1 diabetes occurs when your pancreas can no longer produce insulin. This is usually caused by insulitis, an inflammation in the pancreas. Knowing of CBD's anti-inflammatory qualities, it makes perfect sense that CBD reduces insulitis, thus restoring your body's natural ability to regulate insulin levels. This has been proven in medical studies. [28] In this way, CBD can prevent type 1 diabetes.

The same study takes mice genetically engineered to get diabetes later in their lives, and puts them on CBD treatments.

The occurrence of diabetes drops from 86% to only 30%. [28]

CBD also improves liver triglyceride levels, improved glucose tolerance, and increased insulin sensitivity. Cannabinoids reduce diabetic neuropathy in diabetics resistant to other medications.

Put simply, studies show time and again that cannabis consumers are at much lower risk of contracting type 2 diabetes than non-consumers. [29]

Weight-loss
CBD is shown to raise metabolism, speed fat loss, and lower cholesterol, according to a GW Pharmaceuticals research team based in Britain. [30] Enough said.

Anti-bacterial
CBD as an anti-biotic? You bet! Scientists are shocked at CBD's remarkable ability to kill bacteria. [33] CBD, a natural bactericide, can be consumed to fight drug resistant strains when no other antibiotic will work, and can be used in soaps, cosmetics, antiseptics and creams to fight bacterial infection.

Bone health

Move over, milk! CBD might be the supplement to increase your bone health.

Increased bone mass, decreased bone resorption, and suppressed bone loss are all benefits of CBD. More and more studies are showing CBD as a key method to fighting osteoporosis. [31] In addition to bone maintenance, CBD has also been proven to increase recovery speed in bone-fractures. [32]

Immunity

The function of immune cells is greatly enhanced by CBD. [34] The immunity boost you get from CBD is partially from its anti-inflammatory and anti-bacterial properties, but CBD also boosts white blood cell production and performance. In addition to helping you become healthy, CBD plays a major role in keeping you healthy and preventing disease.

Multiple Sclerosis

CBD relieves muscle spasms, inflammation, and pain associated with MS. [35] Cannabis was used in ancient Greece and China to relieve MS symptoms. [36]

Circulation and cardiovascular health

Scientists have discovered massive cardiological benefits of regular CBD consumption. From improved clotting abilities and circulation, to higher oxygen levels, CBD relaxes arteries, protects vessels from high blood sugar, combats inflammation, and serves to regulate iron levels, all contributing to a healthy heart.

In patients who have had heart attacks, those on CBD endure less heart damage, and a speedier recovery with more and healthier white blood cells. [37]

Digestion and appetite

CBD regulates your appetite. If you tend to eat too much, CBD serves as an appetite suppressant, but in other cases CBD can increase your appetite. It does this by balancing the body's deficiencies and excesses that cause many diseases, but also cause abnormal appetites.

CBD is often used in cancer patients going through chemotherapy to reduce nausea and regulate the patient's appetite. Many of these patients would be unable to eat without the help of cannabinoids. [38]

Psoriasis and skin health

The largest organ on our body also has the most cannabinoid receptors. Of course, I am talking about the skin. Dry skin, dermatitis, and psoriasis, and even more severe afflictions like skin cancer, may be fought with CBD.

A 2013 publication in the British Journal of Pharmacology concluded that CBD has "the potential to be lead compounds for the development of novel therapeutics for skin diseases." [39]

Another recent study shows CBD's promise of fighting malignant melanoma. [40]

Other studies prove the significant effect CBD has on psoriasis, pruritis, and dermatitis caused by allergies.

Allergy relief

Imagine your immune system overreacting to something harmless… just panicking and sending antibodies and triggering inflammation against an invader as harmless as a nut you've eaten, or a flower's pollen. This is essentially what allergies are.

Since most diseases are caused by inflammation, many of our symptoms have root in allergies that we don't even know we have. This is a vicious cycle, in which allergies will cause inflammation, making our tissues more sensitive to potential allergens, which causes more inflammation, and so on.

CBD's natural abilities to reduce inflammation and improve the efficiency of your immune system result in dramatic allergy relief. Get on a regular CBD regimen, and watch your allergies disappear.

Drawbacks of CBD

The side effects of CBD are nearly non-existent. CBD has been proven to be entirely safe in humans. I had to really dig deep to find any potential drawbacks.

CBD may not work for everyone. Every person and every body is different. The benefits discussed in Section 3 are most commonly found to be true, but not unanimously.

There are some people who are allergic to cannabis, but these cases are rare. Nearly all people allergic to cannabis are also allergic to tomatoes and other plants, and *none* of them are allergic to THC or CBD. If you have an allergic reaction to CBD oil, it is most certainly due to its non-active ingredients like the coconut oil it's mixed with. Simply find another source of CBD without your allergy and you'll be able to enjoy the benefits of CBD.

Achieving homeo-stasis

Discussed in Section 2, the way you live your life day to day is what will dictate your overall health. Some habits lead to disease, and other habits lead to health. We can label these habits "good" or "bad" habits, but not in any moral sense. In reality, it's only cause and effect. The habits that lead to feeling good can be labeled "good", and vise versa.

"Bad" habits(effectively, not morally), such as eating junk food, substance abuse, laziness, intellectual distraction(like TV), and spiritual ignorance, will most certainly lead to disease. As these habits become more common in our culture, so does disease.

Likewise, "good" habits, which include emotional maintenance and healthy expression, creativity, healthy eating, positive thinking, meditation, and meditative walking and dancing, will all lead to great health. Do these things every day, and your health will reflect your habits by remaining steady and strong.

CBD supplements can be added to this list of good habits, and will be an integral part of maintaining your mind-body health. I cannot stress enough the benefits CBD provides. It may have the largest influence of all habits on achieving and maintaining *homeostasis.*

How to take CBD

You can take CBD with patches, pills/capsules, or oils. The most common form is CBD oil, a hemp extract very high in CBD, and very low in THC. The CBD oil is then mixed with something to improve its taste, like coconut oil or honey. A few delicious drops of CBD oil under the tongue to enter the bloodstream sublingually one or two times a day will give you all of the benefits discussed in this chapter.

Patches, pills, and capsules are slightly less effective, entering the bloodstream less quickly and less effectively than the oil extract, but will still provide the benefits of CBD. Patches stick on your skin and are absorbed into the bloodstream through the skin, while pills can be swallowed and absorbed through digestion.

CBD can also be taken in gums, shots, vape pens, topical creams, and other means, but are rare and not entirely relevant to this book (even though I regularly use topical CBD ointment for muscle pain relief). Not all of these options provide all of the benefits of CBD. Plenty of information is available online if you want to explore these options.

Important factors in choosing CBD supplements

First, you want CBD from organic and naturally grown hemp. If you're maintaining your mind-body health with supplements that include fertilizers, pesticides, and additives, it kind of defeats the purpose.

Similarly, make sure that your CBD comes from a reputable source that you can trust. Is it pure CBD, from a natural and organic plant? Are the non-active ingredients also organic and natural?

What is the amount of CBD you're getting? Is the mixture you're buying 50% coconut oil and 50% CBD oil? Or is it 80% coconut oil and 20% CBD oil? And remember, there is a big difference between hemp oil and CBD oil. What you want to know is how much CBD you're getting in each "dose".

250mg per ouce is the minimum amount of CBD you should be getting. The amount each person needs on a daily basis is different from person to person, but if a product has less than 250mg per ounce, you're probably getting ripped off.

You will also want to note the THC content. Remember that high THC contents will get you high, and may affect the legality of the purchase, depending on the laws of your region.

Unfortunately, there are many sinister people taking advantage of this new miracle supplement. To turn a quick profit, they may infuse unhealthy ingredients, or use subpar products to begin with. Making a quick and easy buck becomes more important to them than the health of their customers. Such is the world we live in today.

There is no requirement online for sellers to have official testing done to prove their products contains as much CBD as it claims to. There is no requirement to disclose whether a source uses harsh chemicals to extract their CBD, or if they use proper extraction processes. Nor is there a requirement to differentiate between synthetic CBD and natural CBD. [6]

You want a product with a COA, a "certificate of authenticity", to ensure the product you're getting is the product you're selling.

Yet, this is just a warning – a recommendation akin to "buyer beware." CBD is a wonder-supplement, and just like there are bad sources, there are great sources, too. I just implore you to do your homework.

Where to get CBD

I am well versed in the importance of CBD to this world. I have done my homework. I've researched growing habits of providers, tested mixture levels of products, and scanned them for unhealthy additives. I provide the safest source for CBD products on the market at CBDenergetics.com.

At CBDenergetics.com, you can confidently buy safe, pure, properly mixed, properly grown, and properly proportioned CBD products that WILL bring you all the benefits discussed in this book.

Is CBDenergetics.com the only source of CBD products? Of course not. There are other sources, and good ones at that. High-quality CBD, safely and properly grown and mixed, will most certainly provide you all the benefits of CBD, whether you buy them from me or elsewhere. In this free market, if you decide to buy from a source other than CBDenergetics.com, that is fine... just make sure you're doing your homework, and do the research necessary to ensure you're getting a good healthy product. Don't skimp on the research!

Conclusion

The common man's definition of health is a physical lack of symptoms. The common man's solution for his health problems/symptoms is to go to a medical doctor, who prescribes a "medicine" to squash the symptom, but brings other symptoms in tow. The errors of this method are vast.

Health is a balance among our mind, spirit, body, and emotions, and nothing less. To place focus solely on the physical body is to miss a large aspect of health.

Symptoms are not the definition of sickness, but a manifestation. When our mind-body-spirit becomes unbalanced, we invite sickness into our lives, and symptoms follow.

Your health may not be your doctor's priority. His priorities may include pharmaceutical endorsements, increased business, fame, money, or protecting or inflating his ego. At best, even if your doctor is legit and has your health as a priority, he only does what he is trained, and that is prescribing medications to cover up symptoms.

In this book, I have offered a different view, one in which you are enabled to take control of your own health, and experience the best possible life for yourself. Doctors have their place, but we cannot rely solely on them for our well-being. We must take the initiative and begin living healthier lives and forming healthier habits.

Our goal is to experience optimum health, which includes a healthy body, mind, and spirit, with free communication among them, and healthy emotional expression. Adopt these techniques and experience optimum health for yourself.

And finally, we learned of the magical benefits of hemp and CBD. That CBD is relatively unheard of is of great disservice to the world, and I intend to change that. CBD has a growing list of healing qualities and benefits, and should be a part of everyone's daily habits. Visit cbdenergetics.com today!

So, take control of your health! You are a divine being, and should be treated – by yourself – as such.

William Pieper

2016

Bibliography

Introduction & Section 1

[i] http://www.collective-evolution.com/2013/04/11/study-shows-chemotherapy-does-not-work-97-of-the-time/

[ii] http://healthimpactnews.com/2012/30-years-of-breast-screening-1-3-million-wrongly-treated/

[iii] http://www.curenaturalicancro.com/en/75-percent-of-the-physicians-refuses-chemotherapy-themselves/

[iv] http://www.ncbi.nlm.nih.gov/pmc/articles/PMC2360753/

Section 2

[a] http://www.neurosciencemarketing.com/blog/articles/why-expensive-wine-tastes-better.htm

[b] http://www.seattletimes.com/nation-world/a-bitter-shot-for-starbucks-mcdonalds-wins-taste-test/

[c]
http://www.nielsen.com/us/en/insights/news/2009/average-tv-viewing-for-2008-09-tv-season-at-all-time-high.html

[d]
http://www.businessnewsdaily.com/6387-employee-breaks.html

[e]
https://www.youtube.com/watch?v=JcPwlQ6GCj8

[f]
https://www.youtube.com/watch?v=XEX2-m8EabU

[g]
http://www.snopes.com/medical/myths/8glasses.asp

[h]
https://www.youtube.com/watch?v=W80mHIGg9v0

[j]
http://www.rense.com/general62/expl.htm

Section 3
[1]   http://www.drugpolicy.org/blog/how-did-marijuana-become-illegal-first-place

[2] http://www.drugwarfacts.org/cms/Prisons_and_Drugs#sthash.fy14j1Tl.dpbs

[3] http://humansarefree.com/2013/10/hempcrete-best-concrete-is-made-from.html

[4] http://www.hemp.com/hemp-education/uses-of-hemp/hemp-fuel/

[5] http://www.ncbi.nlm.nih.gov/pubmed/22129319

[6] http://www.drugpolicy.org/blog/are-websites-claim-ship-cbd-oil-non-medical-marijuana-states-legit

[7] https://www.drugabuse.gov/about-nida/legislative-activities/testimony-to-congress/2016/biology-potential-therapeutic-effects-cannabidiol

[8] http://www.medicalnewstoday.com/articles/248423.php

[9] http://www.ncbi.nlm.nih.gov/pubmed/22815234

[10]
https://healthyhempoil.com/cannabidiol-pain-relief/

[11]
http://www.tokeofthetown.com/2011/10/cbd_marijuana_compound_has_no_high_but_relieves_pa.php

[12]
http://rheumatology.oxfordjournals.org/content/45/1/50.abstract

[13]   http://www.prnewswire.com/news-releases/can-cannabidiol-cbd-fight-metastatic-cancer-according-to-the-latest-research-the-answer-is-yes-170681736.html

[14]
http://www.ncbi.nlm.nih.gov/pubmed/22198381

[15]
http://www.ncbi.nlm.nih.gov/pubmed/22506672

[16]
http://www.ncbi.nlm.nih.gov/pubmed/850145

[17]
http://www.ncbi.nlm.nih.gov/pubmed/104333

[18]
http://www.ncbi.nlm.nih.gov/pubmed/7028792

[19]
http://norml.org/library/item/introduction-to-the-endocannabinoid-system

[20]
http://www.truthonpot.com/2013/08/14/cbd-may-reverse-brain-deficits-in-parkinsons-alzheimers/

[21]
http://jop.sagepub.com/content/early/2014/09/12/0269881114550355.abstract

[22]
http://www.parkinsonsrecovery.com/cbd

[23]
http://www.leafscience.com/2014/03/05/marijuana-ingredient-may-cure-alzheimers-study-suggests/

[24]
http://psychcentral.com/news/2012/06/07

/marijuana-compound-may-beat-antipsychotics-at-treating-schizophrenia/39803.html

[25] http://www.medicaljane.com/2014/05/28/study-cannabidiol-cbd-may-help-treat-social-anxiety-disorder/

[26] https://projectreporter.nih.gov/project_info_description.cfm?aid=8473835

[27] http://www.sciencedirect.com/science/article/pii/S0091305713002104

[28] http://www.ncbi.nlm.nih.gov/pubmed/16698671

[29] http://norml.org/library/item/diabetes-mellitus

[30] http://www.mensjournal.com/health-fitness/health/the-marijuana-diet-20121108

[31]
http://www.ncbi.nlm.nih.gov/pubmed/213
58974

[32]   http://www.livescience.com/51701-
marijuana-bones-healing-fractures.html

[33]
http://www.ncbi.nlm.nih.gov/pubmed/186
81481

[34]
http://www.ncbi.nlm.nih.gov/pmc/articles/
PMC2748879/

[35]
http://www.nature.com/ijo/journal/v30/n1
s/full/0803272a.html

[36]
https://en.wikipedia.org/wiki/Endocannabi
noid_system#Immune_function

[37]
http://drjakefelice.com/cannabismatrix/201
3/07/10/cannabis-with-cbd-for-heart-
health/

[38]   http://www.beyondthc.com/cbd-and-
appetite/

[39]
http://www.buycbdoilonline.info/2014/06/
cbd-skin-conditions/

[40]
http://www.ncbi.nlm.nih.gov/pubmed/240
41928

Made in the USA
San Bernardino, CA
11 June 2017